HuDGE

What they don't teach us in Medical College!

Dr. Anjali R
MBBS, MS (OBG), DNB, MNAMS

Dr. Naveen R Gowda
MBBS, DPM (NIMHANS, Bangalore),
MD (Hospital Administration, AIIMS, New Delhi)

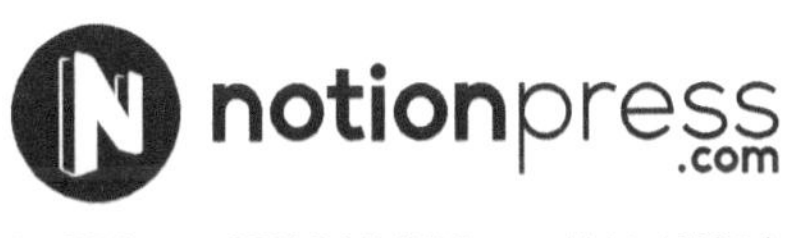

Made with ❤ on the Notion Press Platform
www.notionpress.com

Contents

1. Introduction: Why this book?...5

2. The Problem Statement:
"The Tricky Triad for Medicos"...11

3. Heart of the Problem: Consumption vs
Connect Conundrum...19

4. The Common Denominator:
The ONE Thing We Need to Get Right!...29

5. The Right Tool: How Do We Get It Right?...45

6. What's Your HuDGE?...65

7. The HuDGE Playbook: How to
Improve Your HuDGE?...79

8. The Corporate Constantinople:
Why Should the Corporates Care?...89

9. End of the Road for Health Care Aggregators?...101

10. Start-ups; What Should They Do?...109

11. What Will the Future Look Like?...113

12. Let's HuDGE...125

References...127

CHAPTER 1

Introduction: Why this book?

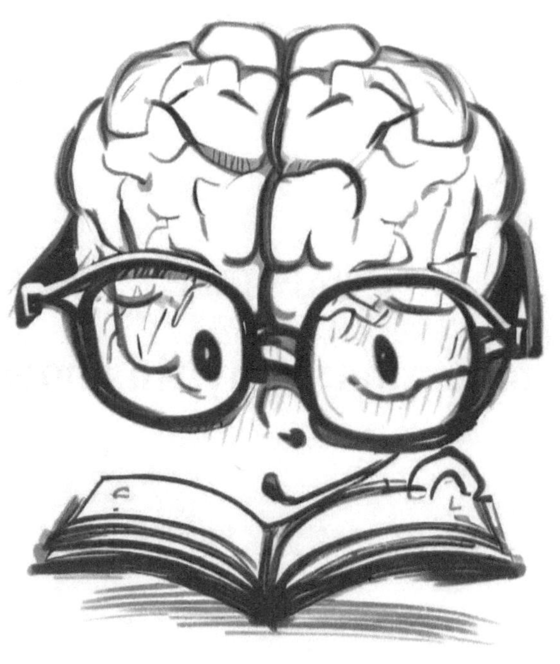

I vividly remember our introductory class by one of our professors when we entered second-year MBBS. We were all gleaming with the achievement of having passed first year MBBS and were already feeling like half doctors.

On a light note, he asked us "What is the biggest challenge for a doctor?" and opened the discussion to the house. We were all supercharged and started thinking hard. We started giving exotic answers like finding cure for cancer, solving India's poverty, free treatment for all citizens etc. Our professor gently smiled and said "The biggest challenge for any doctor is getting patients". The whole class burst into laughter. 17 years down the line, we now see the reason behind our professor's smile.

Medical College has taught us many things, but building a successful practice is not one of them. Call it a science or an art or maybe a combination of both, this remains an enigma for most of us medicos for many years. Be it an apex Institute like AIIMS or any other Medical College in India for that matter, this is an untouched subject. Young doctors, especially in bigger towns and cities are finding it increasingly difficult to build their own practice. It takes them inordinately long for building a practice good enough to earn a decent income.

There are now more than 700 medical colleges in India, about 400 of them having started in the last five years. These colleges are churning out more than 1 lakh MBBS graduates every year. Postgraduate seats have also drastically increased, with more than 67,000 Specialists and about 5,000 Super-specialists passing out every year. However, ironically the National Sample Survey

Organization (NSSO) Health Workforce Survey 2017-'18 has found that 27% individuals with a qualification in medicine – graduation or above – are not active in the labor market, while approximately 4% are unemployed and looking for jobs [1,2,3]. This means 1 in 4 doctors is not practicing or not professionally active. That is flabbergasting!!! Especially when the media, bureaucracy and politicians keep ranting about shortage of doctors.

To make things worse, salaries of young doctors across specialties, especially that of MBBS Doctors has not risen or worse, it has plummeted in few cities. Average salary of MBBS doctors ranges anywhere between Rs. 30,000/- to Rs. 50,000/- per month and the stipend during postgraduate studies in some states is even lesser. There is an increasing narrative around saturation in the healthcare industry and is often cited as a reason for offering low salaries.

On the contrary, with changing demographics and increase in ageing population there is an increase in prevalence of Non-Communicable Diseases (NCDs) like diabetes, hypertension, cancers, chronic kidney diseases among others. According to estimates by Indian Council of Medical Research, 1 in 4 Indians is at risk for NCDs and account for almost 60% of total deaths in India [4]. Rise in disease burden is coupled with economic growth and higher spending capacity which has translated to rising demand for healthcare services and expected to rise further in the future.

According to India Brand Equity Foundation (IBEF), Indian Healthcare industry is valued at around $370

Billion (That's a lot of money!!! Just to give a perspective $1Billion = Rs. 8,000 Crore Approx.) and has been growing at 22% CAGR (Compounded Annual Growth Rate). Medical Tourism has proven to be a cherry on top of the cake, with almost 7 lakh foreign patients coming to India in just the year 2019 and Medical Tourism was valued at $2.9 Billion. India is ranked 10th among the most preferred destinations for foreign patients and is projected to be valued at around $13.4 Billion by the year 2026 (That's more than 1 Lakh Crore Indian Rupees) [5]. Undoubtedly, there is unprecedented growth with many leaders betting on Indian Healthcare to grow bigger than the Information Technology (IT) industry.

Costs of healthcare services has also continued to increase over the years. According to reports, in 2021, India recorded medical inflation rate of 14%, which is the highest among Asian countries. This is also 2.5 times higher than the retail inflation rate of 6-7% in India [6]. That means the cost of medical treatment is increasing faster than the costs of say groceries, vegetables, daily essentials etc. Patients continue to pay more and more with time but most young doctors are earning lesser with time. This appears counterintuitive to the fundamentals of demand-supply mismatch.

So why is our generation of young doctors struggling to build a successful practice despite rising need for healthcare? What are we missing? Well, a lot of free advisors would throw around cliche words like hard work, good behavior, soft-spoken, street-smart, social skills blah blah blah as "mantras" for building a successful practice. But we all know that these superficial jargons don't help much. Not everybody who is soft-spoken has a successful practice and vice versa. Successful doctors come in all shades and profile.

What can actually help us is a tool or a technique to objectively assess our practice, give us insights on our weaknesses and help us improve & strengthen our practice. HuDGE is an effort in this direction. It's a tool built on fundamentals of behavioral economics, combined with data from rigorous market research. In short, HuDGE is a tool that can help young doctors build and sustain a successful practice.

To keep it practical and relevant, there are no jargon or fancy B-school lingos. Just plain simple English that we doctors understand. So, let's get started!

CHAPTER 2

The Problem Statement: "The Tricky Triad for Medicos"

"A problem well stated, is a problem half solved"

– Charles F. Kettering

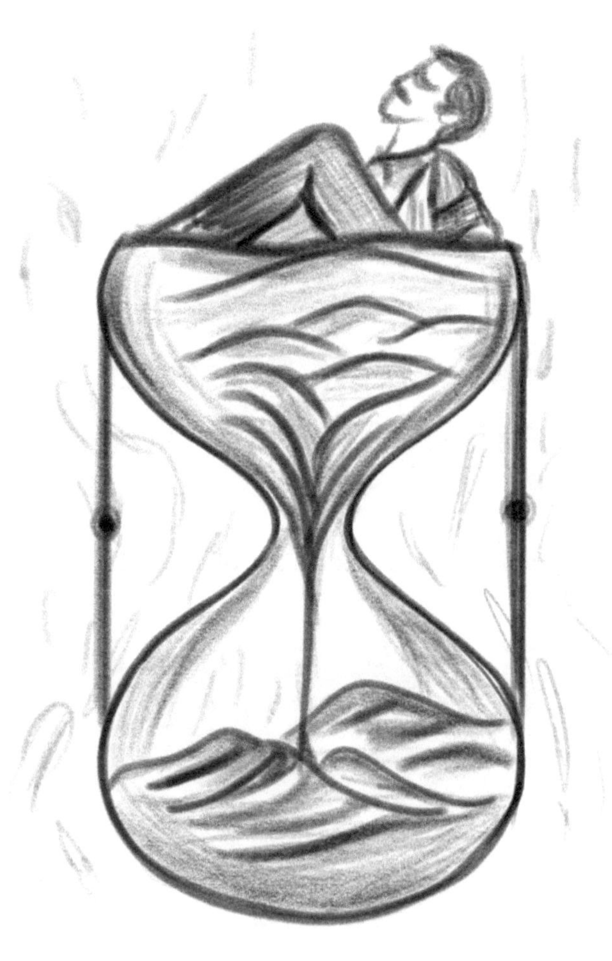

As young struggling doctors we already have enough on our plates, unless we have inherited a flourishing nursing home or hospital, a luxury most of us don't have. So, in the middle of all that we are going through it is easy not to see the nuances. It is sometimes frustrating to feel stuck and not being able to progress. To address any problem, we first need to define it well. So, lets understand our problems a little more. Most of the problems that we medicos face finally boils down to 3 distinct yet interrelated challenges that we call "The Tricky Triad".

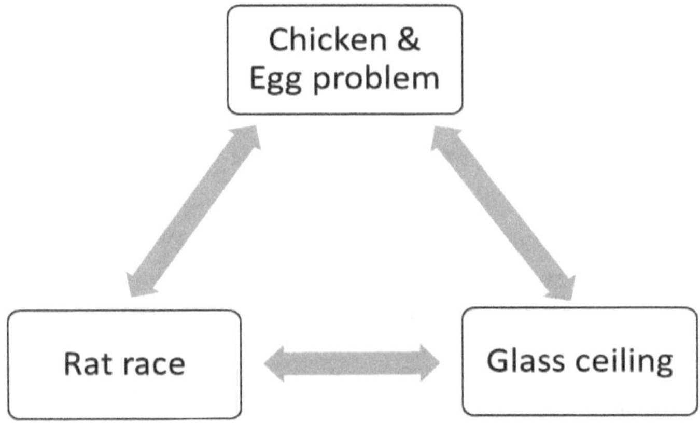

Figure 1: The Tricky Triad for Medicos

1. The Chicken and Egg problem:

Having set-up one's own practice is one of the important signs of progress for doctors. It is not only important for professional growth but also personal wellbeing and satisfaction. Working under someone in a hospital or corporate set-up is a stop-gap arrangement most of us do till we feel confident of hitting out on our own.

However, setting up own clinic involves cost. Right from renting out a place, getting basic furniture, equipment and hiring support staff, we would need both upfront capital investment and running expenses to subsequently maintain it.

This is definitely a challenge in the initial few years till our practice picks up. It may take a few months or sometimes a couple of years to build a practice good enough just to pay-off the rent, bills and salaries. It is only after our patient footfall reaches a certain level that we actually make a sustainable income for ourselves. We will have the same challenges even in group practice, polyclinics and corporate hospitals. Some corporate hospitals offer a minimum guarantee salary for a year or two which gives some leeway, but the pressure is always on and catches up pretty soon. This often becomes a reason for many of us to postpone our plans of being independent consultants and we half-heartedly drag on working in junior positions.

This is the common "Chicken and Egg problem" wherein we can't kick start our independent practice till we have enough patient base and we will not have enough patient base till we kick start our practice. This gives rise to the second problem.

2. The glass ceiling:

Not knowing where to draw the line and when to start independently is a very tricky situation. Most of us end up on the back foot playing a safe game by working under some established senior doctors. This provides safety net and sort of a cocoon or comfort zone. Financial apprehensions drag this even further and most of us would probably prefer remaining assistants. We all have seen many doctors continue to work as assistants even during their late 40s. This phenomenon is more glaring in the surgical disciplines.

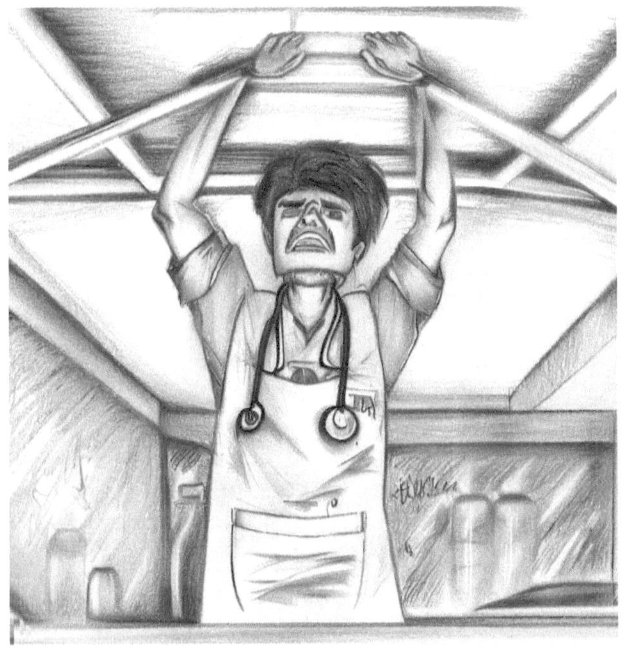

This is the infamous glass ceiling. You cannot really see it, but it is definitely there and it takes a lot to break beyond it. The ones who have an established practice usually do not like new entrants coming in and taking-over their patients and rightly so. They may not actively resist or stop the newer entrants but they will certainly not give things on a platter. None of us would do it either. This pushes us towards the third problem.

3. The rat race

When the hard reality of glass ceiling hits, most of us take respite in studying further by getting into fellowships, training programs etc. This behavior is based on an assumption that more the degrees we have more patients will come to us, pushing us into a perineal rat race, not really knowing where to stop.

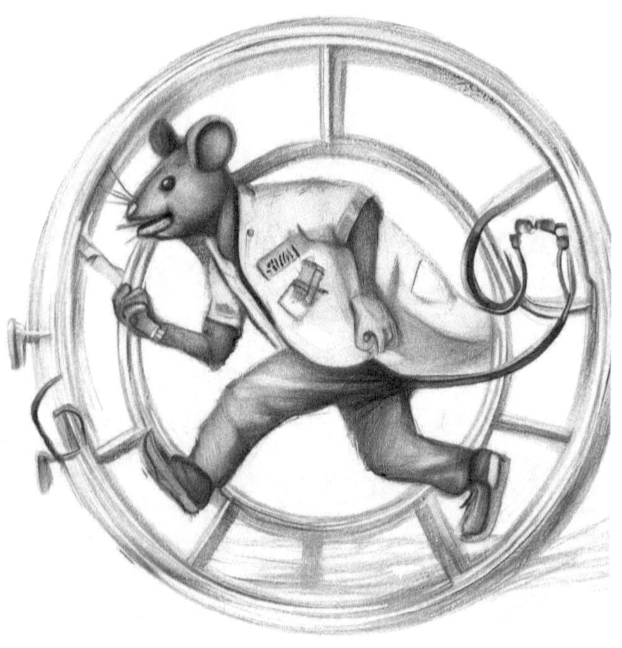

Besides, most of the fellowships and training programmes do not pay stipend or salaries. This further adds to financial insecurity and yet the rat race continues. With passing time, it only becomes more and more difficult to get into mainstream and the vicious cycle continues.

So, when we take a step back and see, most of the problems we are facing like low salaries, difficulty in finding the right job, almost-never ending student life, not being able to settle down, can all be explained by the vicious cycle set in by the Tricky Triad. Doctors who manage to break out of this vicious cycle actually start doing well.

So, why are we stuck in this vicious cycle? We need a broader understanding to answer this question and that takes us to the next chapter.

CHAPTER 3

Heart of the Problem: Consumption vs Connect Conundrum

"What consumerism really is, at its worst, is getting people to buy things that don't actually improve their lives."

– Jeff Bezos

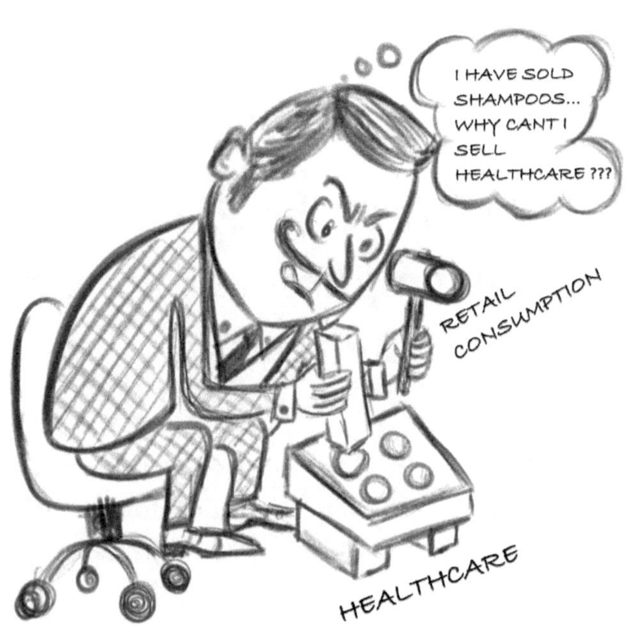

I HAVE SOLD SHAMPOOS... WHY CANT I SELL HEALTHCARE ???
RETAIL CONSUMPTION
HEALTHCARE

Before 1980s majority of healthcare services was provided by the Government sector. People had to travel to the big cities with medical colleges even for basic healthcare amenities and go abroad in case of complicated procedures. That is when some of our visionary doctors took the lead and stood up to the challenge. They built private hospitals to provide the much-required tertiary care to the masses. With economic liberalization in 1990, growing population, increasing spending capacity and rising middle-class, the private hospitals started doing financially very well.

When any sector appears lucrative, it is natural for private investments to flow in. That's how many investors and investment funds started funding and opening hospitals with primary objective of giving good returns to investors and thus started the era of corporatization.

Corporatization has brought in the much-required funds to bring in cutting edge technology and provide best-in-class services. Some of these companies are now public and listed on stock exchanges which has helped them in raising more funds for expansion and also given an opportunity to the common people or the retail investors to become part of this growth story. With time more and more investments started flowing into building hospitals since it appeared as a very good investment option, to the extent that currently more than 70% of healthcare services are provided by the private sector.

Now let's understand how these market forces function. Most of the big-ticket private investments are going into secondary and tertiary care to building hospitals and other healthcare facilities. The average revenue per occupied bed per day ranges anywhere between Rs. 35,000 to Rs. 50,000 depending on the type of the hospital, location and disease profile. The average operating cost per bed ranges anywhere between Rs. 10,000 to Rs. 20,000 per day per bed depending on the type of the hospital. This is just the cost of running and the hospital is burning this money whether there are patients or not. Cost of marketing, sales, administrative overheads among others are incurred on top of these operating expenses.

Besides, majority of consultants in corporate sector are engaged on Fee-For-Service model and therefore their fees can be yet another addition on top of operating expenses. So, we can safely assume that any hospital would need at least around 30-40% occupancy in order to just sustain, as they cannot afford to lose investor money. Currently the whole system is geared up to put people in hospitals as the very business model demands ensuring sufficient occupancy and cash flows to even sustain.

That brings us to the fundamental question of how to get the patients to the hospital in order to maintain the requisite occupancy. Like it or not, there is a definite cost incurred in bringing the patients up to the hospitals. This is referred to as the customer acquisition cost (CAC). Often it is neither measured nor reported by most of the hospitals as it is not easy to calculate.

To understand this better let's first look at the factors that influence a patient's choice of hospital. For the sake of discussion, let's exclude the minuscule section of know-it-all, internet frenzy patients. For the majority, the journey mostly starts with a felt need which is followed by discussions with their trusted social circles. Then, depending on the recommendations, past experiences or hearsay, the patients first consult a doctor within their family circles or a local doctor who is easily accessible. Most of the minor ailments are managed at this level. In case in-patient care is required, the treating doctor would most of the times, refer the patient to his colleagues in higher centres. It is pertinent to note that most of these referrals are in the name of doctors, unless it is one of the Apex centres or government institutions.

Interestingly, >80% of private providers are smaller family-run, mom & pops hospitals or nursing homes. Many of these have been built by doctors who start with a clinic and expand as they build their patient base and therefore, they do not depend on any form of marketing or sales teams. The fact that they exist in large numbers and continue to function implies they are financially doing well.

On the other hand, most of the corporate groups have full-fledged marketing and sales teams with the ultimate objective of driving patient footfall. The marketing and sales guys would want us to believe that they are primarily responsible for patient footfall (because they need to keep their jobs!) but that does not seem to be true. The impeccable emphasis and heavy dependence of most of the corporate hospitals on recruiting and retaining "Star consultants" implies otherwise. Therefore, we can say that the patient footfall in any hospital is predominantly dependent on their doctors' ability to draw patients.

A significant proportion of patients who come to hospitals would have been referred from the doctors in the community. However, conventionally primary care has been seen to have low margins and often seen as not profitable. This could possibly explain very little private investments done at community levels. This approach of investing on building hospitals was okay till the time there were fewer players in tertiary care. With more and more foreign investments flowing in, new brands emerging, competition at tertiary care level is getting heated. This has prompted more expenditure on the marketing front, wherein the corporate hospitals mostly end up hiring *"Marketing Experts"* from other sectors, who are nowhere related to healthcare.

Their first instinct would naturally be to copy and paste the marketing strategies that have worked well in other domains. Replicating time-tested techniques from other fields appears to be a good idea from the outset. They have been largely successful in replicating the marketing strategies used for selling soft drinks, tooth paste or chips for marketing Entertainment or Fintech products. Then why can't they use the same strategies in Healthcare?

Well, there's a big catch. The very premise of marketing in say FMCG, retail or entertainment is to increase consumption, that is to make the consumer buy more and in-turn spend more. Unfortunately, the same principles are being applied to healthcare, which translates to making the patients spend more. Increasing consumption has taken precedence over building connect which is a fundamental flaw.

In the process, the good old trust-based referral channels with personal touch appears to have taken a backseat as approaches used by FMCGs (Fast Moving Consumer Goods), retail marketing, entertainment industries are fast creeping into the boardrooms and lingos of corporate hospital chains. Recent remarks by the honorable Chief Justice of India regarding the growing trust deficit about medical services in India [1] is partly a reflection of this fundamentally flawed approach.

These factors create what we call "The Corporate Chakravyuha". Let's use the principles of Game Theory to understand this better. When there are two or more players, over a period of time they would have reached an equilibrium, wherein everyone gets to survive. For example, if you take Pepsi and Coke, both compete in the same space of carbonated drinks and both have the same pricing. They have kind of achieved an equilibrium wherein both get to make money without cutting the price of their products.

But when a new player comes in with newer offerings, the equilibrium goes for a toss, as we have seen in case of India's telecom industry. Most of the players were charging us a handsome money for calls, SMS and they had some form of equilibrium. But when Reliance Jio entered the market and offered free services, they disrupted this equilibrium and forced other companies to cut their prices. This led to a cut-throat business war amongst the companies but finally benefited all of us, the common users, big time.

Now when we extend this analogy to the private sector in Indian Healthcare, we see many new brands entering the same space of secondary and tertiary care. Heated competition disturbs the prevailing equilibrium amongst the incumbent competitors. One player spending more money on patient acquisition automatically prompts the others also to up the ante, for maintaining the minimum required occupancy and utilization. This cost is finally passed on to the patients.

Therefore, we can say that rising customer acquisition cost which is a fallout of lack of community connect, is one of the key contributors to overall rise in treatment costs in hospitals. These culminate in decreasing trust levels which in turn makes patient acquisition harder for these hospitals and the vicious cycle continues. The unfortunate part is that, unlike the telecom sector where increasing competition benefited the common users, it is just the opposite in healthcare. These have neither benefited the patients nor the doctors.

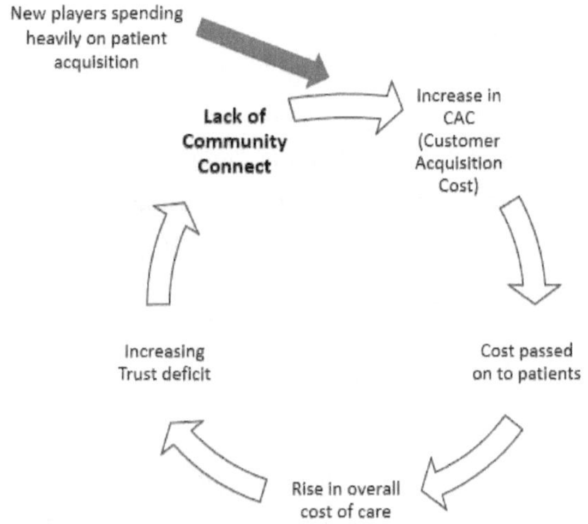

Figure: *The Corporate Chakravyuha*

Gradually, some players have come to realize that primary care is the Gateway for hospital business and have started opening clinics, but with limited success. Again, this is because of the consumption versus connect conundrum. They are missing the very fundamental elements.

Okay that is the problem of hospitals, right? How is it relevant to us as practicing doctors? Well, we are an integral part of the ecosystem and the market forces also have an influence. Most of us find it difficult to get out of the rat race which is based on a wrong assumption that merely having more degrees/fellowships will automatically get us more patients. Most of us assume that once we become super-specialists with many degrees and fellowships, we will get a swanky office in one of these Hospitals and the hospital will get us more patients. Well, that's not how it works! In fact, the hospitals bank on their doctors' ability to pull patients. Since we do not invest our time and efforts in building our own patient base early on, we do not have the escape velocity to get out of the tricky triad.

So, when we step into the real world, we realize it takes time to build our patient base and some of us end up trying shortcuts like depending on marketing agents, middlemen and aggregators to get patients. But most of the times these don't work or even worse, backfire. The patients that these middlemen or aggregators promise are often diverted from some other doctors. They will divert your patients if they get higher commissions from elsewhere, making these modalities highly unreliable and unsustainable.

The hospitals are definitely looped in the consumption versus connect conundrum and finding it harder to bring in more patients. Many of us are also missing the picture and end up flocking the corporate chains, hoping to get started!

So, what are we missing? What is that one thing we need to get right? That brings us to the next chapter.

CHAPTER 4

The Common Denominator: The ONE Thing We Need to Get Right!

"You only have to do a few things right in life and not get many things wrong".

– Warren buffet

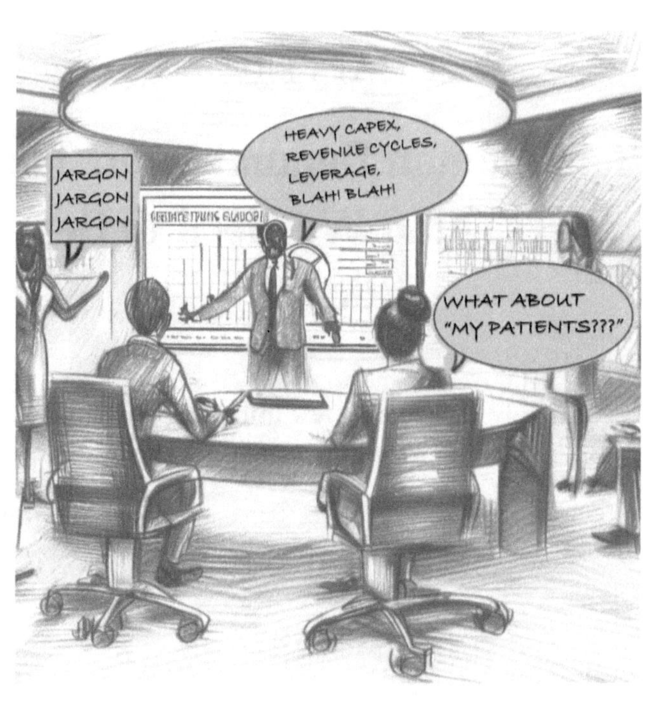

JARGON JARGON JARGON
HEAVY CAPEX, REVENUE CYCLES, LEVERAGE, BLAH! BLAH!
WHAT ABOUT "MY PATIENTS???"

As young doctors we need to acknowledge that our time is a valuable and finite resource. How and where we invest our time today will determine our future trajectory. As Warren Buffet rightly pointed out we only need to get a few things right in life. So, what is that ONE THING that we need to get right? What is that one common denominator that really matters to be successful?

To derive the answer, let us first understand how Indian healthcare industry functions, who are the different stakeholders, what are their challenges and what is it that they are looking for? It is pertinent to remember that almost 70% of health care services in India is taken care by the private sector. They do not get any form of financial support from the government per se and need to sustain by themselves. We should not waste time on never ending, emotionally biased moral debates that fit the narrative for dramatization and illogical vilification. Rather, lets objectively understand things based on data, facts and then draw logical and realistic inferences.

Let's begin with the Hospitals. Whether it is nursing homes, standalone hospitals or corporate chains they all need to pay bills, give salaries, repay debts, pay taxes like any other business entity. The thumb-rule in Hospital Planning says we would require an upfront capital investment of anywhere between Rs. 60 Lakhs to Rs. 1 Crore per hospital bed. This varies widely depending on the cost of land (it varies widely depending on the location), disease profiles treated, proportion of critical care beds, equipment, facilities and other support services.

For example, if we plan to set-up a tertiary care 50-bedded hospital with say 10 ICU beds, 2 Operation

Theatres, 1 Cath Lab, blood bank, Central Sterile Supplies Department (CSSD) or Theatre Sterile Supply Unit (TSSU), Medical Records Department, Medical Gas Supply Systems, Laundry, Generator back-up, just to list down some of the required facilities, it can cost us an upfront investment of anywhere between Rs. 30 Crore to Rs. 50 Crore. This money can come in as debt (loan) or equity (by giving shares to investors) and either way there is a cost to this capital. Then comes the cost of running this this 50-bedded facility which can cost us anywhere between Rs. 4 Lakh to Rs. 5 Lakh per day.

So, naturally any hospital or nursing home will invariably have to ensure a sufficient patient footfall, bed occupancy and utilization of their services. In short, they are looking for a strong patient base. This reflects clearly in their recruitment policies as well. As doctors, we get a fixed salary (although it may not be much) as long as we continue to work as a Duty Doctor, Resident, Registrar, Junior Consultant or any such position where we do not have rights to independently admit patients.

When we are ready to upgrade to the position of an independent consultant with rights to admit our own patients, we start with something called a Minimum Guarantee pay. This will be given for a year or two depending on the hospital. This runway is given so that we can build our patient base. After this short period, we will mostly be asked to work on fee for service basis. Depending on the type of hospital and their financial appetite just around 15 to 25% of consultants would be on minimum guarantee pay at a given point in time. The rest of them are engaged on fee for service basis. *Simply put, we will earn proportionate to the number of patients we can bring in.*

When we study the size and distribution of hospitals in India, it is interesting to note that more than 80% of the hospitals are less than 50 bedded capacity [1]. Report of Sub-Group-IV of Expert Committee on Enhancing Resource Investment in Health (ECERIH) commissioned by the Government of India states that Corporate Hospitals account for just around 1% of total hospitals in India and 67% of corporate hospitals are clustered in just 8 big Indian cities [2]. Corporates have always struggled to establish themselves in smaller cities and towns, where the small hospitals and nursing homes run by local doctors certainly fare better. Most of them start a clinic and as patient footfall picks up, they steadily upgrade into nursing homes and hospitals. Undoubtedly the unorganized sector dominates.

Let's move on to Diagnostics, which broadly includes labs and imaging services. According to HDFC Securities report, Lab industry is valued at $9.5 billion dollars and is growing at a rate of around 11% every year in India [3]. Let's try and understand the fundamentals of the Diagnostics business and how it runs.

Diagnostics, just like hospitals, is a capital-intensive sector. The equipment are expensive and rapidly advancing technology means that they need to keep on investing on upgrading as well. Expenditure is broadly into two categories: Capex, which is the money required to create the facility and Opex is the money required to run the facility. Starting a Diagnostic centre from scratch would require space, licenses, regulatory approvals and compliances, followed by machinery and equipment, reagents and manpower to run it. Besides, going for outright purchase of these equipment will lock-in large sums of money, which not many can afford.

So, over the years the many labs have come up with newer ways of getting the equipment like "rental purchase" wherein they need not pay the full amount upfront. This, of course, has a catch. They will get the equipment for free or a discounted price, but will have to buy the reagents to conduct the tests from the same company. The diagnostic centres will also have to give a guarantee for purchasing certain minimum quantity of reagents every month. That means whether they actually conduct that many tests or not, they will have to pay that minimum money to the equipment/reagent companies. Therefore, it only makes sense for the diagnostic centres to ensure volumes or risk losing money.

Interestingly, the average profit margin in labs ranges anywhere between a whopping 50 to 80%. We have ourselves negotiated Business to Business (B2B) prices with an average discounted price of 70%-80% from a NABL accredited reference lab. Just to give an example, Thyroid Function Tests (T3, T4 and TSH) costs anywhere between Rs. 800-Rs. 1000/- in local labs and around Rs. 500/- on e-pharmacies/ aggregators. We had negotiated the same tests for Rs. 150/- on B2B basis with a reference lab. And guess what, this margin further goes up with increasing volumes.

How is this even possible? Well, it is pretty complex and a big industry in itself. For ease of understanding, as one of the lab guys explained to us, let's take the example of hormone assays. Each batch can run anywhere between 500-1000 samples depending on the machine. Whether the labs run just 10 samples or 600 samples in a batch, their fixed costs will remain more or less the same. Based on marginal costing, it only makes sense to run more samples and to get more samples they offer deep discounts to their B2B clients. Hence the huge profit margins.

No doubt everybody wants to put their hands into this pot of gold. Right from big business houses like the Reliance group, Adani group to the retail investors, there is growing interest with huge investments flowing in. In fact, Diagnostics are one of the important revenue sources even for hospitals which is why we commonly see that any hospital of a reasonable size would have its own in-house Diagnostic facility. This is reiterated by the fact that 37% of the labs in India are hospital-based [3].

Diagnostics sector saw a bull-run during peaks of COVID-19 pandemic. Most of the labs registered a sharp increase in revenue and profit margins. However, as the pandemic recedes, there has been a steady decline in volumes. This market correction was expected as the high volumes were largely tests related to COVID-19 which have now fallen drastically. Besides, newer players entered during the pandemic which has now intensified the competition and even the legacy companies have not been able to get back the growth seen before the pandemic [4].

Despite huge investments, the corporate lab chains have not been able to make significant headway. According to the HDFC Securities report, the four major players –

Dr. Lal Path Labs (DLPL), Metropolis Healthcare (MHL), SRL Diagnostics (SRL) and Thyrocare Technologies (TTL) – together account for just around 6% of market share. If we include other regional chains, their combined market share is again just around 16%. Dr. Lal Path Labs, being one of the oldest chains and a market leader, gets 40% of its North India revenue from Delhi-NCR alone. Clearly, the corporate lab chains are predominantly seen in metro cities and larger cities and not so much in tier-2 and tier-3 cities. The local standalone centres are the dominant players, accounting for a whopping 48% of the total labs in India [3].

Most of us would wonder how are these small, local, stand-alone labs managing to dominate and dodge the big "organized" players backed by heavy funding. The answer partially lies in the fact that 55% of the lab business reportedly comes from referrals from local doctors and 35% of the business comes from walk-ins which also are mostly from some form of indirect referral channels. Barely 10% of business comes from Corporate clients. The industry is definitely fragmented with dominance of unorganized sector, which makes it difficult for the corporate groups to scale [3].

The imaging sector consists of high end, expensive equipment like CT, MRI, Doppler, Ultrasound, X-rays among many others. It is definitely capital intensive with high cost for both starting and running imaging facilities. Let's assume we plan to install a 64-slice CT scan and a 1.5 Tesla MRI machine, both being descent, mid-range specifications by current day standards. A 64-slice CT scan machine can cost anywhere around Rs. 1 Crore and a 1.5 Tesla machine can cost around Rs. 7.5 Crore in case of outright purchase [5].

Then there is the cost of land, construction, AERB approval (for CT machine), power back-up among others at the time of setting them up. Then comes the running cost that includes manpower, electricity, consumables among many others. There is an interesting study by Saho et al on lifecycle costing and breakeven analysis of MRI [5]. It is important to remember that there are many variable factors like the financing of equipment, salaries of staff, pricing of scans and other recurring expenses that can vary widely between centres and therefore different break-even points.

So, let's not get bogged down by numbers or complexities. When we run some simple math [6], we can find that in order to just break-even i.e make just enough revenue to avoid losses, the imaging centres will require to do at least 200-220 MRI scans and 300-320 CT scans per month when they charge an average price of Rs. 6000-Rs. 7000/- per MRI scan and Rs. 1000-Rs. 1500/- per CT scan. Even if we take 25 working days in a month, *the imaging centres will have to do 8-10 MRI scans and 12-14 CT scans per day in order to sustain.*

Yet again, it would not be surprising to see a skewed distribution of these facilities, with most of them concentrated in and around metro cities. In fact, if we go by the media reports, the MRI market in India is shrinking at around 3% per annum and the government turned out to be the biggest buyer [7]. This means that private buying has gone down despite the high growth rate of healthcare industry per se. This is probably because investors are not sure of getting the required volumes to break even, which in turn is possibly because they do not understand their consumer behavior at grassroot level.

Now let's move on to pharmaceutical companies which are yet another major stakeholder. To get a better understanding of this sector, let's take a life-cycle approach and understand how different stages right from drug discovery to market entry are functioning. It takes more than $100 million (Approx Rs. 800 Crore) to bring a new drug into the market [8]. Interestingly, about 40% of this cost goes towards finding and recruiting patients for clinical trials [9]. In case of any delays in patient recruitment, a Pharma company can lose around $1 Million (About Rs. 8 Crore) every passing day [9]. This problem is so pertinent that there are companies in the US which make the process of patient recruitment smoother, efficient and less expensive. High profit margins in the Pharma Sector have been both a reason for its success as well as frequent criticisms about undue profiteering. Being one of the oldest industries, the incumbent players are considered to be very powerful with strong lobbying capabilities.

Indian Pharma sector has many interesting paradoxes. IBEF report states that the Indian pharmaceutical sector supplies over 50% of the global demand for various vaccines, 40% of the generic demand for US and 25% of all medicines for UK. According to the Indian Economic Survey 2021, the domestic market is expected to grow 3 times in the next decade. India's domestic pharmaceutical market stood at US $ 42 billion in 2021 and is likely to reach US $ 65 billion by 2024 and further expand to reach US $ 120-130 billion by 2030 [10].

India has 1/6 of the world's population and yet only about 1.4% of clinical trials happen in India[11]. Despite a double-digit growth rate and tremendous potential in Indian markets, it would be surprising to know that some of the MNCs, which are dominant players in the US and Europe, are finding it difficult to grow in India. Pfizer closed down two of its facilities due to falling demand, Danish company Lundbeck exited Indian markets, Novartis and Eily Lily sold their marketing and distribution rights to Indian companies and laid off their Indian employees [12]. All these companies are formidable forces in their respective countries but have not been able to penetrate the Indian market beyond the tier 1 and metro cities. They have not been able to replicate their success in the West. What could possibly be the reason?

The answer is not that simple though. There are many factors ranging from regulatory framework to Intellectual Property rules. However, one factor stands out to be significant and that is, *who holds the decision to buy the drugs?* The United States healthcare is largely insurance driven and the prices of drugs are negotiated centrally which are then procured in bulk by the providers/ hospitals. The UK has NHS, which is funded by the taxpayer money and most of their procurements are centralized. In simple words, the western countries have a clear-cut laid out structure and process for procurement which makes it easier for these companies. They just need to manage these key decision makers for their business.

On the contrary, in India most of expenditure incurred on outpatient basis happens out-of-pocket by the patients themselves. The patients' decision is in turn decided by the prescription of their doctors. Therefore, there is no well-defined predictable and controllable channel for marketing and sales. These MNCs practically will have to approach all the important doctors in every city if they want to stay in business. Besides, managing to succeed in one city/place does not guarantee success even in the neighboring towns. They have to work ground-up in every single city, which is an operational nightmare for these companies who are used to working in controlled & structured environments. This is one of the major reasons why the MNCs have resorted to outsourcing the marketing activities to Indian pharma companies who understand the landscape better.

Okay how is any of this information relevant to us as practicing doctors? Let's connect the dots and find out. It is interesting to see that scalability is a significant challenge for all corporate entities; be it hospitals, labs, imaging centers or multi-national pharma companies, with most of them struggling to enter smaller cities. This is certainly not because of lack of investments. It is because Indian Healthcare is largely hyperlocal with the unorganized/ informal sector being in a dominant position. This appears like the David and Goliath story where David despite being small prevails over the giant Goliath. So, how is this even possible?

Let's first understand what is unorganized sector and how is it different from its organized counterpart. In simple words, entities in unorganized sector mostly operate locally, they are run mostly on small investments by single owners and cater to demands of the local population. Generally, there is little data/information about them and therefore makes them less predictable with very limited scope for control. On the contrary, data on business and finance of entities in formal/organized sector is largely available making this sector easier to predict and control.

This simply means that if the same corporates operated say in the US, they will have direct access to say 300 million (30 crore) consumers since the majority of the healthcare industry is in organized sector. This makes it easy to scale. But when informal sector dominates, the market is fragmented and just because a hospital/ lab/ company succeeds in one city, it doesn't guarantee same success in another city/place. Therefore, scaling up in unorganized sector is always challenging. This also means that any policy change by the government or heavy investments by big corporations will not have the same impact in Indian healthcare as compared to the US or other western healthcare markets.

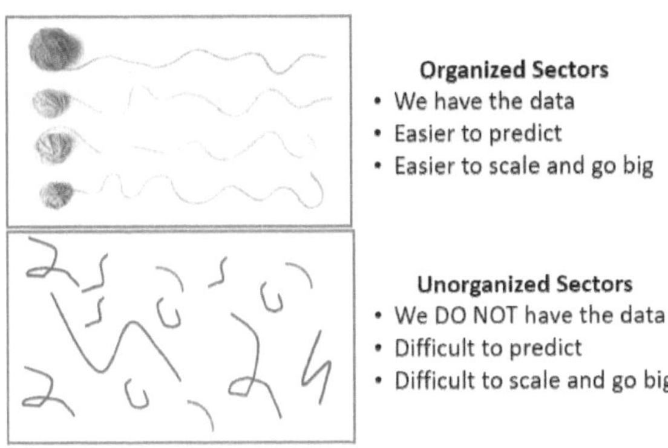

Figure 1: Organized vs Unorganized Sector

This is happening because the entire hyperlocal system in Indian Healthcare completely revolves around strong Doctor-Patient relationships and bank on the trust of the local communities. Even the paramedical service providers like physiotherapists, nutritionists, occupational therapists, home care nurses, clinical psychologists among others are also largely dependent on referrals from local doctors. *Currently the entire system is heavily dependent on local doctors who have a good patient base.*

Finally, let's talk about the most important stakeholder, the patient. Let's try to decode the psychology behind patient's choices. Social proof or social validation plays a very important role in determining the patient's choices of their doctors. This means that people tend to choose the options already chosen by other people with a presumption that if so many people have chosen it, it must be right. Therefore, social proof is also often referred to as herd mentality.

The famous "busy restaurant syndrome" is a good example of social proof. In this experiment when people were given choices of an empty restaurant, partially filled restaurant and busy restaurant, most of the people chose to go to the busy restaurant assuming that if so many people have chosen it, it must be good. Based on the same analogy, patients also prefer doctors who already has a good patient base.

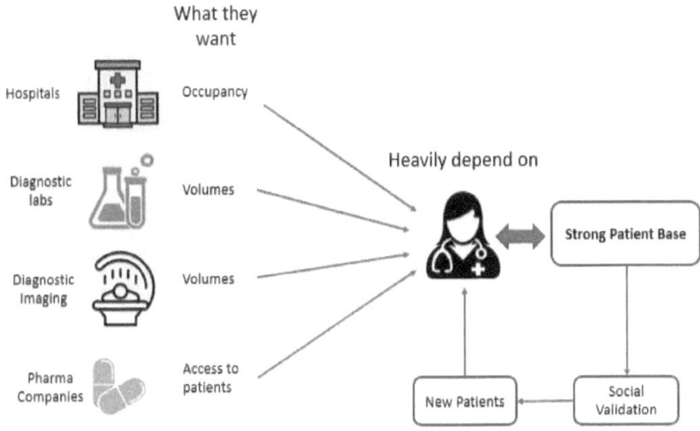

Figure 2: *Doctors with strong patient base as Gateway to Healthcare*

This is both a wonderful opportunity and a social responsibility that we enjoy as doctors. We as practicing doctors are practically the gateway for our patients to the rest of healthcare because of which we are in a strong position to get the best for our patients from other industry players. Clearly, if we have to invest our time and energy in getting that *ONE THING* right, it should be *BUILDING OUR OWN PATIENT BASE.*

How do we do that? Do we have any tools or techniques that can help us? That brings us to the next chapter.

CHAPTER 5

The Right Tool: How Do We Get It Right?

"In God we trust, the rest of you bring data"

– Edwards Deming.

In God we trust. Rest of you marketing guys, bring data!!!

– That's just us!

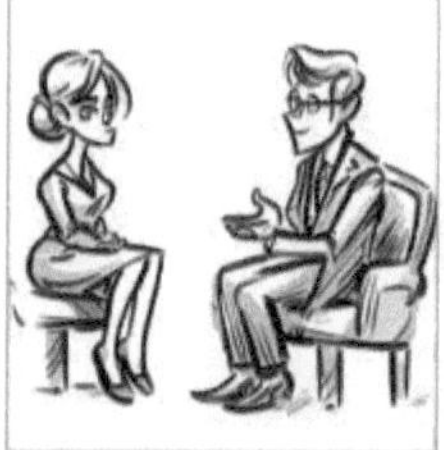

WE'VE SPENT TONS ON DIGITAL MARKETING ... RESULTS ???
WE'VE RUN CAMPAIGNS...

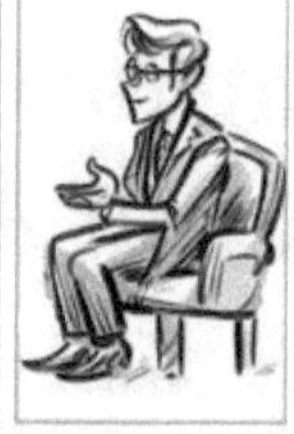

YOUR AD CLICK RATE IS 65%

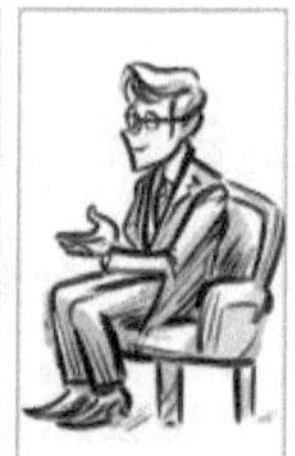

AWESOMENESS METRICS IS UP 40%

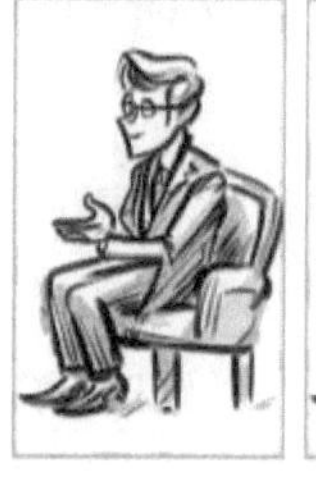

YOUR COOOL QUOTIENT IS UP 36%

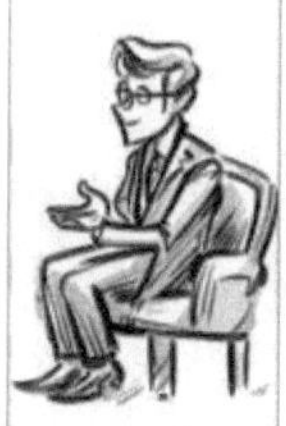

AND YOUR B.Y.O.P SCORE IS RECORD HIGH AT 100%

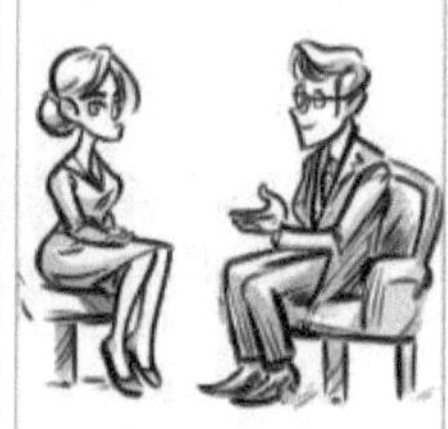

WHAT IS B.Y.O.P !!???
WELL... BRING YOUR OWN PATIENTS !!!

Okay, we now know that THE ONE THING we need is OUR OWN PATIENT BASE. But how do we achieve this? We need to smartly invest our precious time and effort on techniques that can give us higher dividends. Not to mention, most of us also do not have the luxury of extra money. So, all the more a good reason to find the right tool!

Of late there are many self-proclaimed *"marketing gurus"* who are trying to profess so called marketing strategies to doctors. If we look closer, they are essentially repackaging case studies on marketing techniques being used for Fast Moving Consumer Goods (FMCG) (it's a swanky term for commonly used stuff like toothpaste, soap, facewash or sugar water), retail, entertainment finance etc, without paying attention to the nuances and differences in healthcare.

In all fairness, none of the fancy B-school guys would have ever seen a patient so they can't really understand the finer details, nuances or what it actually means to see patients. Besides, we should also remember that any marketing activity should not cross the fine lines or boundaries set by the moral code of ethics by the Medical Council of India. We need to look at evidence and data before deciding on which technique or tool suits us the most. Technically, we should be asking "In God we trust. The rest of you marketing guys, bring data!!!" Let's now analyze the different options.

Marketing in itself is a very broad subject with many different schools of thought. The good old conventional marketing are time-tested approaches which have worked really well in other sectors. For the ease of understanding, these marketing campaigns can broadly be seen as either Above The Line (ATL) or Below The Line (BTL). This is a gross oversimplification, but it helps to get a broad overview.

Above The Line campaigns are mostly mass communication channels like newspapers, television, radios, billboards, hoardings etc. It is difficult to target a specific profile of customers with these approaches and is generally intended to generate curiosity, introduce a new product or reinforce the existing brand image. Below The Line campaigns are slightly more subtle, personalized and targeted. They include door to door campaigns, events, tele calling, mass emails, bulk SMS, bulk Whatsapp campaigns among others. There are many successful case studies for these approaches and they undoubtedly continue to be the mainstream marketing strategy for many industries, ranging from retail, finance, entertainment etc. However, their effectiveness in healthcare is highly questionable and not tested or proven.

Let's start with ATL (Above The Line) marketing. How effective can front-page newspaper ads, big billboards/ hoarding or radio ads be? Honestly, this is a big question for the marketing world itself as it is very difficult to measure their impact. Let's look at it from healthcare point of view. One of the most important aspect in healthcare is the "Information Asymmetry". This means that patients, more often than not, are not sure what they want in the very first place. There is a significant knowledge gap between the providers/doctors and the consumers/ patients.

Let's compare it with other sectors for a better understanding. When people want to buy groceries, books, clothes or electronics items, they already know what they want. It is only a matter of choosing between different available options in the market. So, bombarding them with ads on television, radio, billboards, signboards etc makes sense. On the contrary, in case of healthcare, the patients are aware of their problems but are not sure what to do about it. That means random, swanky advertisements about some high-end equipment or procedures, would not mean much for them. Leave alone patients, many medicos might not be aware of such things.

The other important factor is that Healthcare in India is largely hyperlocal (as we discussed in the previous chapter) with each practicing doctor having a "Catchment area" from where most of their patients come. That means most of our patient base would be from the town/district that we practice in or at best neighboring districts. Therefore, ATL approach doesn't make sense as it is expensive and unlikely to be of much benefit.

Talking of Below The Line (BTL) techniques, most of us would have experienced the excruciating pain and frustration of being subjected to spam calls, cold SMS and bulk WhatsApp. There was a meme on WhatsApp (Figure 1) recently which shows how BTL marketing can go wrong! Jokes apart, if anything, these only create sense of mistrust for the brands which are doing it.

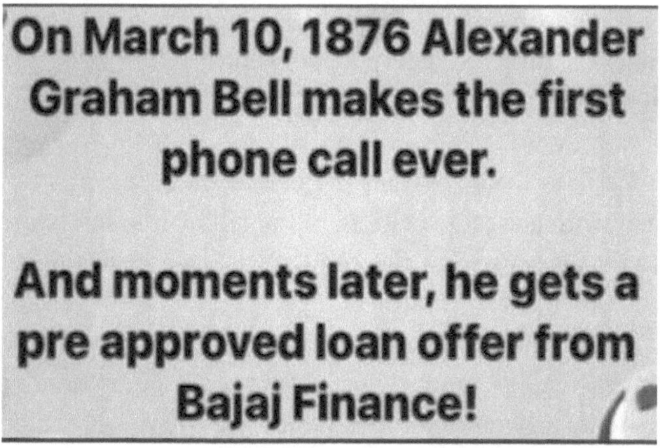

Figure 1: Cold Calls gone wrong! (A meme on WhatsApp)

If any healthcare company/ hospital creates such an impression with Cold calls or cold SMS, that's practically the end of the road since it can create serious trust issues about such entities/hospitals. As for conducting events or door to door campaigns, they are pretty expensive and require efforts. Besides, these are more suitable for one-time campaigns like music concerts or elections. Since public memory is short-lived and there is little recall or memory reinforcements, events or door to door campaigns can fizzle out really fast. Therefore, BTL too doesn't help much in building our own patient base.

Let's move on to a trending modality of marketing that is digital marketing. We often encounter marketing agencies who toss around terms like social media, leverage, Search Engine Optimization (SEO), Ad words, etc. They promise to get more patients by providing greater visibility on digital ecosystem. Of course, they charge quite handsome money for this job. So, let's find out whether this modality is worth investing in.

Let's first understand how this works. Let's say a mobile phone company comes up with a new model. They obviously want as many people to know about their new product and to reach out to their potential customers. So, they hire a digital marketing team, who will post advertisements on leading platforms like Google, Facebook, Twitter, Instagram etc. While posting these Ads, they can choose their target audience by adding details like age group, geographical location, gender, professional background among many others. The more specific these details, the more precise will be targeted marketing.

Now these Ads are displayed specifically to the chosen target population, therefore increasing the chances of selling the product. The platforms like Google, Facebook, Instagram etc get paid every time a viewer clicks on these links. How much of these clicks actually gets converted to sales depends on the respective product website and the platforms get paid even if no sales happen. In short, they get paid for generating leads.

This is a booming business in itself which has created humongous companies like Google and Facebook. Just to get a perspective, Google's (parent company alphabet Inc) valuation stands at a whopping $1.3 trillion (that is roughly 10 lakh Crore Indian Rupees) [1]. Google's revenue reportedly in the year 2022 alone was $ 280 Billion dollars [2] which is more than the annual budget of many countries. Reportedly, more than 80% ($224 Billion) of this revenue comes from online advertisements [2,3]. Likewise, majority of revenue for other platforms like Facebook, twitter, Instagram etc also come from online advertisements. Needless to mention, these platforms are next to magical when it comes to targeted marketing which is evident from their revenues.

But when it comes to their success in India, the findings are quite contrary and very interesting. Google's annual revenue from Ads from India is reportedly around Rs. 25,000 Crore ($ 3.1 Billion). This is barely 1.3% of Google's total global revenue from Ads [4]. This implies that digital marketing isn't delivering the same results in India and is definitely not as effective when compared to the west. Many digital marketing guys would argue that India's internet penetration is way less compared to the developed countries and attribute it to low effectiveness of digital marketing. Let's check some basic facts and run some simple math to see if this is true.

India has a total population of 140 Crore people. More than 83 Crore people have access to internet. The average monthly data consumption is 16.4 GB per user [5]. Let us compare this data from India with that of OECD (Organization for Economic Co-operation and Development) which is a group of 38 countries from across the globe, most of them doing economically well. OECD countries collectively have a population of 138 Crore. 91.5% of them have access to internet. The average monthly data consumption for all OECD countries put together is about 8.38 GB per user[6].

So technically *an average user in India is consuming double the data consumed by an average user in OECD countries.* Even if we take the cumulative total of data consumed by all the active internet users, *India consumes about 30% more data than all OECD countries put together!*

So, the argument of lower internet penetration and usage in India clearly fall flat. Therefore, it is clear that digital marketing is not as effective in India compared to other countries.

Just because people have access to internet and are using it well does not necessarily mean they will spend/buy online. This is also evident from the fact that YouTubers (People who have YouTube channels and put content on it) from India earn far less than YouTubers in the US and 70 other countries! One of the main reasons is the low CTR (Click Through Rate) in India [7]. CTR is the number of times an ad is clicked divided by the number of times it is shown. This means that Indian viewers are far less likely to click on Ads and consequently less likely to buy from these online Ads.

So why should we doctors really care? Well, all these numbers simply mean that the average revenue per user for any digital platform is way lesser in India compared to the US, Europe or any OECD countries. In simple words *Indians are far less likely to buy or spend based on these online advertisements as compared to people in US or Europe.* That means it is not an effective option and naturally we should be skeptical about investing in Digital Marketing.

But the Digital Marketing dudes will try to hard sell by saying it is growing fast blah blah. Let's look at some more data. Whatever little is happening in Digital Marketing is largely from other sectors with 38% coming from FMCGs, 30% from e-Commerce, 5% from automotive and healthcare doesn't figure anywhere close [8]. Again, good enough reason not to go for it. Now the marketing dudes will try the last trick in their book, FOMO, Fear of Missing Out. They will try to convince us by saying that other doctors have started using it.

Let's try and find out with a simple exercise. If we randomly search for star practitioners in our respective cities on the internet, we can see they hardly have any reviews. Even in tech-hubs like Bangalore and Hyderabad which are known for techie-crowd, best of the doctors will have far less reviews than a famous restaurant. In smaller cities, we may not even be able to find these star practitioners on the internet, forget reviews. These again support the fact that internet is not the first choice when people look for doctors, they rely more on their social circles.

On top of this, healthcare in India is hyperlocal. Most of our patient base comes from same or surrounding districts, leaving little scope for digital marketing. Therefore, *as practicing doctors, digital marketing is not of much use for us and it is not worth spending money and time on it.*

Most of us would wonder what could this possibly be due to? What makes India different? After an elaborate literature search, it appears to be predominantly due to cultural aspects. Quite often India and most of the oriental cultures are said to be low trust markets. This means that consumers in these markets are less likely to trust new companies or sellers and therefore less likely to give them a try. This cultural fabric and factors are so strong that it has humbled even giants like McDonalds and Kellogg's who have come up with Indianized products like the Mc Aloo Tikki and Upma respectively. Li et al in their research article outline many possible explanations for this phenomenon. The very fundamental fabric of individualism versus collectivism, power distance and uncertainty avoidance could explain a lot of this consumer behavior [9].

	India & Oriental cultures	Western cultures	Influence on consumer behavior	What it means for Digital Marketing
Individualism Vs Collectivism	Predominantly collectivism	Strong individualism	Consumer decisions influenced by social groups in Oriental cultures	Word of Mouth takes precedence in oriental cultures. Reason why Digital Marketing is way less effective in India compared to west.
Power distance	Significant. Strong hierarchy and Information Asymmetry	Relatively lesser.	Consumer decisions require social validation in Oriental cultures.	
Uncertainty avoidance	Higher with more risk aversion	Lesser	Willingness to try new products lesser in oriental cultures	Digital marketing being impersonal & faceless, less likely to be trusted.

Table 1: *Cultural fabric, Consumer Behavior and Digital Marketing*

That brings us to the healthcare aggregators and middle-men who openly profess and promise to bring-in more patients. Let us first understand that what aggregators do, how they function and how they make money? They work on something called the e-commerce business model. They act as platform/middle-men between sellers and buyers.

On one side, they will have many products or services from different sellers and on the other side they have buyers. The buyers get the same product at their doorstep often for a cheaper price. This attracts the tech-savvy crowd and provides a good bargaining capacity to the aggregator. They now talk to the sellers and negotiate discounts and sellers are happy to give it as they need not bother going out searching for buyers.

Retail aggregators like Amazon & Flipkart, fashion aggregators like Myntra, cab aggregators like Ola and Uber, insurance aggregators like policy Bazaar, likewise, there is a long list of successful aggregators who also have the tag of unicorns (companies which valuation of more than $1 billion). Please note that many of them are not yet profitable and burning cash as they are giving out huge discounts for retaining their customers.

Let's now try to understand the consumers behavior through the steps involved in the buying cycle. The very first step is awareness of the need. The consumers should know what he wants. This is followed by assessment of options where the consumer compares the different options available in the market based on certain parameters like specifications, cost etc. This is followed by risk-benefit assessment, wherein the consumer weighs the risk vis a vis the benefits of buying. Once he is convinced about all these, the buying happens. Depending on the experience, the customer decides whether to buy again from the same seller or not.

In case of groceries, electronics, toiletries, fashion stuff etc. "awareness of need" is very clear. The consumers exactly know what they are looking for. The aggregators also provide useful comparisons between different options at their fingertips. Consumers often know the price at which the same product is available in regular shops as well. The benefit of convenience and discounts outweigh the potential risk of getting a substandard product. Simply put, getting substandard grocery, defective mobile phone or damaged books cannot kill anyone. At worst consumers will stop buying from the platform.

Now let's analyze the same buying cycle with reference to healthcare aggregators. As discussed in previous chapter, Information Asymmetry plays a key role in healthcare and the very first step of awareness of need itself is often not there. Patients just know they have a problem, but are not sure what the problem is and do not know what to do about it. The next step of comparison between options is out of question because patients most of the times do not have even the basic information and understanding. Also, they need to be sure that the available options are of comparable quality or equally good. This also is not the case in healthcare. Most often they do not know on what parameters to compare doctors, hospitals, labs, pharmacies etc. The only thing patients really want when they are ill, is to get well.

Moving on to the third step of risk-benefit analysis. *The risk of choosing a wrong option far outweighs the benefits of any amount of discounts or convenience in Healthcare.* Consulting a totally unknown doctor from a totally different city can be a very eerie experience for most patients. Likewise choosing options other than the ones suggested by their treating doctor also has high perceived risks. The very nature of information asymmetry doesn't make healthcare conducive for aggregators and they seem to have missed-out on the very process of decision-making by patients. (More on that in chapter 9).

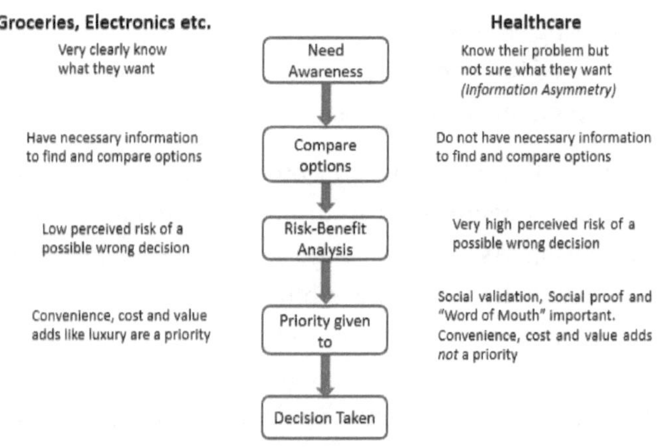

Figure 2: Consumer Decision Pathway Healthcare vs Others

Now let's look at some market research data to find out if the aggregators can be of any use to us. One of the major challenges for any aggregator or any app for that matter, is retaining users/ customers. Market research by different agencies found that the average 7-day app retention rate is said to be barely around 5-6% and 30-day retention rate was just around 1-2%. This simply means that if 100 people download an app, only 6 of them continue using it after 7 days and only 2 of them continue to use it after 30 days [10]. These numbers vary depending on the sector, but by and large the average retention is pretty low [11, 12]. No doubt Customer Acquisition Cost (CAC) has become the noose around their neck, as many of them bleed cash and struggle to sustain.

Aggregators in other sectors like retail, news, entertainment, fin-tech etc, depend heavily on discounts, push notifications on their apps and bombarding users with calls, SMS and WhatsApp. They use these techniques to repeatedly get back the users on their apps. A survey report found that 82% of people who buy online reported that they buy online because of big discounts [13]. This is a tight spot for aggregators because they can't stop the discounts as they will lose users, on the other hand these discounts are not financially sustainable. Push notifications are yet another thing they use. These are basically the notifications that we keep getting on our smart-phones. It turns out they aren't that effective either, with barely 3-5% CTR (Click through Rate). That means if 100 people are sent push notifications on their phones, barely 5 of them click/open them [14]. Then comes the cold calls, mass SMS and bulk WhatsApp, which are, the least to say, irritating.

Healthcare aggregators are no different and are trying to do it the same way as other aggregators. The law of reversed efforts in psychology states that the harder you try to sell something to someone who is not totally convinced, the lesser are the chances they will buy-in. If anything, they will only get more paranoid. Healthcare is a very personal and sensitive matter. When healthcare aggregators resort to cold calls or spam SMS/ emails mimicking aggregators in retail, they may actually end up losing ground.

Besides, retention rate for healthcare apps also is barely 2% which is extremely low by all standards. When the aggregators are themselves struggling to retain their users/patients, how can they get us more patients? So, if any aggregator or middlemen are promising to bring-in more patients, they are bluntly lying! For all we know, they would be diverting some gullible patients from some other doctor on the platform and it would only take a little more commission to further divert our patients even before we know it. Therefore, *aggregators and any other middle-men are definitely a big NO in our journey of building our own patient base.*

Based on these discussions, we now know that conventional marketing, digital marketing or aggregators cannot really help doctors build one's own patient base. Then, what will actually work? How do we achieve this?

Okay, so let's put the pieces of the puzzle together to figure out the solution. India basically being a low trust market, word of mouth or social approval play a vital role in success of any new product or service. People won't try new things unless they hear about it from their trusted social circles. In case of healthcare there is information asymmetry, where patients heavily depend on their doctor's advice for any decision and this is compounded with need for risk mitigation wherein patients would not want to take risks with a totally unknown or new provider.

These factors make Indian healthcare largely hyper-local which is strongly rooted in trust and building relationships. In short, a trusted doctor influences all health-related decisions and is practically the gateway to healthcare for their patients. They command a position where they can Nudge their patients to make the right choices. This, my friends, is THE HUMAN NUDGE aka HuDGE.

HuDGE is the capacity of a doctor to build her/his own cohort of patients, be the trusted go-to expert for all their healthcare needs (big or small) and the extent to which the doctor can nudge her/his patients to make the right choices or decisions.

HuDGE is therefore the tool of choice for us, young doctors, for building our own patient base.

If we pay attention to the doctors who have a very successful practice, they will invariably have a very strong HuDGE. In fact, most of us would wonder what the marketing teams in corporate hospitals actually do. Well, apart from the usual marketing stuff that doesn't work, they are largely engaged in finding out Star practitioners in and round their hospital's localities. They practically map out all the clinics and have a fair idea about the patient footfall in each of these clinics. They then use this information to negotiate financial terms with these successful practitioners to create patient referral channels for their hospital.

This is known by different names like referring physician connect, GP engagement, practice buyouts etc. So technically speaking even the corporate marketing dudes are banking on doctors with a strong HuDGE (although without acknowledging it!). In fact, stronger our HuDGE, more will be our pay package and doctors who have a strong enough HuDGE are even offered partnerships in hospitals. That is the power of HuDGE.

HuDGE is something we all clearly see and strongly feel. As doctors we all understand that HuDGE is THE TOOL OF CHOICE. Most of us keep wondering about this obvious yet enigmatic tool. In order to use it effectively we first need to understand how HuDGE works. Let's use the concept of "Social Capital" from behavioral economics to understand HuDGE.

"Social Capital" essentially means our relative value in the society. Just like "financial capital" in some way reflects our position in the society and enables us to get things done, Social Capital provides us the access to social groups which has many inherent benefits. The difference is that unlike Financial Capital which is easily measurable and is more transactional, Social Capital is more subtle and runs on emotions and trust. From evolutionary point of view, humans have lived in social groups as it gives them easy access to resources and information which makes life easy. Now what does this have anything to do at all with HuDGE? Well, a lot actually!

The moment we enter medical college, we automatically earn Social Capital as we are seen by our social circles (family and friends) as resourceful people. Remember "Information Asymmetry" is a major determinant in healthcare. When it comes to Health, everyone wants to be in safe hands. As seen previously, the risk of a wrong decision in matters of health is perceived to be very high and therefore increases dependence on experts/ professionals.

So naturally as doctors, we are often seen as people with the right information by our social circles. Most of our relatives, friends or their friends, neighbors etc consult us not necessarily for treatment, but to just know who is the best doctor to consult for their conditions. In fact, as doctors we ourselves bank on our fellow medicos to find out the right specialists for a particular condition when it is beyond our purview.

The fact that as medicos or doctors we can understand the medical conditions better itself makes us useful. The fact that we also have the necessary information, network and means to connect the patients to the right specialist just adds to our usefulness and therefore adds to our "Social Capital". To be part of a social group each individual will have to bring something to the table. They will have to add some value that others in the social group find useful.

That brings us to the "Word of mouth". Word of mouth is basically people exchanging information they have about a place, person, product or anything of some significance, in return for some social capital. That means when people have trust in a doctor, they will be forthcoming to share that information with their social circles because that makes them appear resourceful in their social groups.

Social capital automatically brings with it a strong sense of trust. This forms the very foundation of HuDGE as our suggestions and advice as doctors are often valued, sought and followed. This is what actually helps us to build our own patient base and in turn a successful practice. So, how do we know what is our HuDGE? Let's check it out in the next chapter!

CHAPTER 6

What's Your HuDGE?

"You can improve only what you measure"

– Peter Drucker

When you <u>don't</u> know your HuDGE...

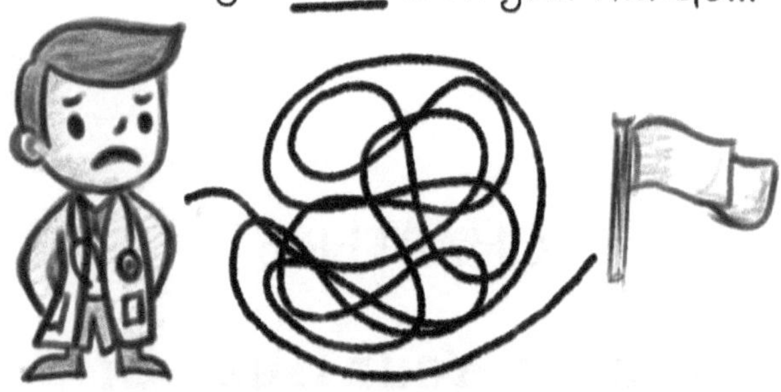

When you know your HuDGE...

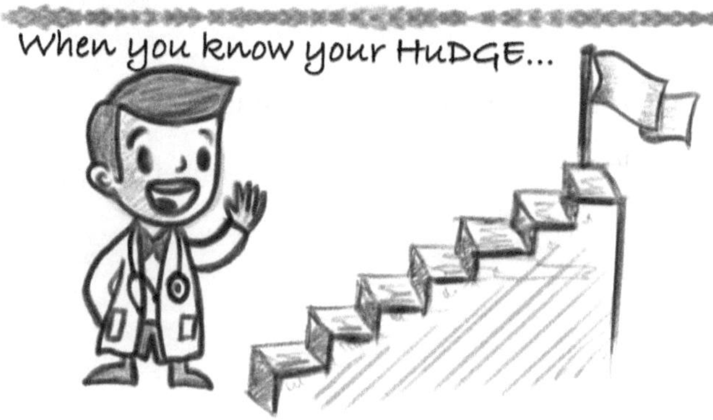

We now know that HuDGE is an effective tool and an assured way to build successful practice. In order to improve anything, we first need to know where we stand and therefore, we need to objectively measure our current status. HuDGE per se is rooted in building trust and meaningful relationship with our patients. Well, a lot of us would already know this. The difference is that it has never been measured and analyzed objectively. So, this made it seem like successful practitioners were successful maybe because of their backing, their backgrounds, their luck factor etc. It is kind of taken that only a few can be as successful. That is definitely not the case. Our research over the last seven years with more than 10 successful projects (one of them being funded by AIIMS intramural grant) culminating in around 18 international publications, combined with behavioral economics and market research, has shown that we can objectively measure, assess and systematically improve our HuDGE.

HuDGE has three components: Continuity, Clinical Outcomes and Word of Mouth. Each of these components has three elements, with a total of nine elements. These nine elements are built into an algorithm which is used to calculate our HuDGE. Let's understand each one of them.

I. Continuity:

The first component, Continuity, is a basic requirement to build our HuDGE. It means we are actively involved in our patients' journey and assisting them in every step of decision making. Okay, that kind of seems vague. How do we measure it exactly? Well, how good our continuity is, can be measured with three elements.

1. How many families rely on you as single point of contact?

Most of us take this for granted, and at times even avoid as we move higher in the specialization ladder. It is becoming increasingly common to see superspecialist struggling to practice as they do not have their own patient base and it definitely takes time to build one. These families are your cohort and you are generally the first go to doctor for them in case of any queries, big or small. They may not essentially seek curative treatment from you always but they will definitely ask you to recommend the best doctor for their condition.

Therefore, irrespective of whether you are a fresh graduate, specialist, super specialist or even from preclinical or paraclinical/diagnostic branch, your cohort will always look up to you for the first advice. This is the social capital you have earned being a doctor and is an invaluable asset in your professional life as well. And it generally starts with your own family, friends, relatives and extended families of relatives. As people get to know you, your friends, their families and their friends and their families start associating with you depending on how approachable you are.

Even after you refer them to other specialist for their conditions, A lot of them would even come back to you for a second opinion, reassurance and guidance. Now that my friends, is your patient treasury, the very foundation of your professional life and career. Most of us would have never bothered to quantify or measure this aspect. You would be surprised to see the progression of your patient treasury when you actually measure it. This is where HuDGE as a tool can help you.

2. What is the follow-up rate or attrition rate of your patients and how good is their compliance or monitoring?

Follow-up rates would definitely vary with the disease condition and specialty. However, continuity of care remains the common thread, irrespective of disease condition or specialty. It is equally important that patients who come to you for the first time continue their link with you for achieving better clinical outcomes. This is an important part of Continuity of Care spectrum.

Follow-up need not necessarily be only after you treating them. Your patients coming back to you just to update about their journey or other consultations, in itself is a part of strong follow-up. Also, patients with chronic diseases or non-communicable diseases would be maintaining well on medications but definitely require longitudinal follow-up and monitoring. This is the second element that can be longitudinally measured with HuDGE.

3. How many doctors are there in your referral network and how many patients you refer and how many you get as referrals?

Being single point of contact for many families also means that you would be referring many of your patients to your seniors or colleagues of other specialties. Cross referrals are a very important aspect of continuity. Most of you would already be doing it, though informally and mostly in an unorganized fashion. When you refer any of your patients to any other doctor, it generally makes sense for that particular doctor to refer the patient back to you, for better continuity and vice versa.

Because there are no formal channels and since it is usually not done systematically, patients dropout somewhere midway, hampering continuity. This eventually culminates in poorer clinical outcomes, increase in disease burden and therefore the patients loose. The doctors also loose as their patient base get eroded with time. HuDGE helps in measuring and streamlining this vital element.

II. Clinical Outcomes:

Building a strong patient base requires continuity, which in turn is strongly determined by the clinical outcomes. Yet again, when patients do not come back to you either for follow-up or monitoring, it is generally presumed that the patient got better. But many studies have proven otherwise. Loss to follow-up is a major impediment especially in chronic diseases requiring long-term treatment and monitoring.

Objectively measuring clinical outcomes is not just important to you as a doctor but is equally or more important for the patients themselves. It is important that your patients see those small little improvements in their health status every now and then. It is only when they see some impact or improvements of the first few steps, will they continue the requisite treatment, monitoring and follow-up with you. It is also extremely important to reinforce the trust with your patients which will be beneficial for all.

Most of you will have only cross-sectional information about your patients which provide only snapshots. Therefore, leaving very little room or scope for actually measuring clinical outcomes. This is happening again largely because we do not have any system in place to enable us. HuDGE can help in measuring clinical outcomes through three elements:

1. How well are you able to longitudinally track health status of your patients?

This is especially relevant for specialties dealing with chronic illnesses. It is an important aspect of disease prevention and keeping your patients out of hospitals. There are various scientifically validated, objective tools that help in some way to quantify the disease severity, risk score and even prognosis. For example, HAM-D (The Hamilton Depression Rating Scale) for depression, Framingham Stroke Risk Score (FSRS) for stroke, Indian Diabetes Risk Score (IDRS) for diabetes risk and many more. But the question is how often, how effectively and in what proportion of your patients are you able to use it? Well, most of you wouldn't really know the answer for this because you would not have measured it.

So first you need to pick the right tool for the right disease condition for the right set of patients and second you also need to longitudinally measure it. There are numerous risk assessment scoring systems available. HuDGE being a holistic technology can assist you in choosing and using the right tool for your patients from time to time.

2. How many Emergency Room (ER) admissions were avoided?

I am sure this is an element that none of us would have ever measured. The very premise of treating patients is to keep them out of hospitals and to minimize the need for emergency care. Sporadic events like road traffic accidents, falls are of course not predictable and should not be considered under this element.

Known case of cardiac diseases, diabetes, hypertension, kidney diseases, mental illnesses among many others are supposed to be under monitoring of a doctor. If follow-up and monitoring are done meticulously based on validated risk assessment, emergency room visits can be minimized. Even more important is that you calculate it and your patients actually know how many ER visits you have prevented for them.

3. In case in-patient care was required, were you in loop during admission and after discharge?

This is an important element that indirectly reflects the trust your patients have on you and also the strength of your referral network. As a primary treating doctor, it is good to know the updates on your patients in their clinical journey. Your patients in times of need will look up to you hoping you may have some control on what is happening with their treatment. Information is the fundamental prerequisite for any form of control and patient journey or patience course through the healthcare system is no exception. When you refer your patients to other specialists already in your referral network, it becomes easy to get information/updates on your patients' condition. This again most of you would not have measured.

III. Word of mouth:

This is a combined output of how strong your Continuity with your patients is and how aware are your patients about their clinical outcomes. Word of mouth has always been one of the most powerful tools in the evolution of human civilization. It has the power to make or break empires, governments, brands and companies. It is an important aspect of people's social life.

Word of mouth is an essential component of social capital. As we have seen in chapter 5, we as human beings are fundamentally wired to increase our social capital as it gives us many benefits like access to key resources. Social Capital largely has three parts viz; Cognitive resource, Structural resource and Relational resource. Each individual in a social group has to bring something to the table in order to be part of the group and invariably would be bringing in one of these three resources. Cognitive resource is largely valuable/useful information, structural resources are broadly physical assets like money, house, vehicles etc. and relational resource is having trusted network of people willing to help when required.

Cognitive resource is commonly used by people in their social groups. This means people who are privy to important and useful information that many others don't have, can get access to structural resources and relational resources by sharing this vital information with their social circles. This is especially relevant wherever there is information asymmetry and wherever wrong information can be potentially hazardous. This means wherever people do not have authentic information on vital things, they rely on their relational resources that is social circles and peers, for the right information. Their social circles would be equally keen on sharing their cognitive resources as they get more relational resource in return.

In simple words, in case of health care, people who would want to know the best doctor for their condition would first ask their trusted social circles and their social circles would be equally keen to share this information as it further strengthens their mutual trust. This also means that people would not want to risk their relational resource or trust with their peers about information they are not sure of. Simply put, people will give your reference as a good doctor and spread through word of mouth only when your initial set of patients and their families trust you. I am sure this is something most of us would have never thought of, forget measuring it.

Word of mouth can be broadly measured with three elements:

1. In what proportion of your patients do you involve their families in providing care and educate them?

There is increasing evidence that says any disease condition needs to be seen through the Bio-Psycho-Social model. This means any disease or illness will have biological component, psychological component and social component. As Medicos we are well trained in managing the biological aspects and rarely touch upon the psychological aspects and almost always forget the social aspects. If you pay enough attention, you will actually notice that right from disease risk factor, delayed diagnosis, poor medication compliance and eventually poor outcomes are linked to the social circumstances of the patient in some way or the other.

As doctors we certainly cannot solve all their social compulsions. But we certainly can engage their immediate family members or caregivers and make them part of the journey. This not only reinforces faith and trust of the family in you, but it also improves clinical outcomes. By doing this you are practically equipping them with cognitive resources that they will be more than keen to share with their social groups in return for relational and structural resources.

Simply put, once they have the trust on you, they will be more than eager to suggest you as the preferred doctor to their social circles because this also helps your patients' families to appear helpful and resourceful in their own social circles. They also want to be thanked and remembered by their social circles for referring them to a good doctor like you. That is how my friends, word of mouth spreads. Therefore, it is important to measure how well you are engaging and educating your patients families.

2. How many of the new families who got associated with you, were referred by your existing patients and their families?

This is one of the easier ways to measure how strong is the word of mouth. Wherever people do not have the necessary know-how or information or objective yardsticks to measure, they heavily depend on their social circles for credible information. Let's take for example purchase of gold or property vis a vis purchase of groceries, electronics or any other things of daily need. When it comes to gold or property, people do not always have the necessary information to compare different options and decide which one is the best. Besides, the risk of a wrong decision is pretty high. Of late BIS hallmark for gold and local authority recognition papers for properties have somewhat bridged the information gap. But still word of mouth plays a very strong role in these decisions.

On the other hand, people mostly have the required information to compare and choose from different available options for say things of daily needs. Also, a wrong decision could barely cost them anything. Therefore, neither do people find it important to ask or share their opinions about these things and therefore role of word of mouth may not be as much. Knowing how many of your new patients were referred by your existing cohort of families is a good reflection of how well "Word of Mouth" is working for you.

3. What proportion of your patients or their families know about your achievements from time to time?

This one is definitely not easy to measure but pretty effective. Your patients mostly do not understand complicated disease names and medial jargon. What appeals to them is the narrative of how you played an important role in making someone's life better. These narratives are largely colloquial which is easy for common people to understand. Human mind works best on contrasts and comparisons which can be used while explaining the disease conditions, treatment or prognosis to patients and their families. We all grasp better when we can quantify and compare unfamiliar things like medical conditions to familiar things like currency, percentages, proportions etc.

It is very important for the patients and their immediate caregivers/ families also to quantify the improvements. This is an extremely important trust building measure and is one of the major determinants of medication compliance. This gets better when they share these narratives with their social circles. Therefore, showcasing your achievements in terms of the impact you have had provides the much necessary content for the "Word of Mouth".

Alright, we now know that HuDGE can actually be measured through its three components and total of nine elements. Now you would obviously think whether you can measure it by yourself. Of course, you can, but it can turn out to be time consuming and laborious. On the other hand, you can use our algorithm to measure it from time to time.

To start with, you can interact with the algorithm through simple questions and answers. We are working on automating this process also with our algorithm doing all the work for you. Check out chapter 12 and the QR code, use your unique access code at the bottom of the page and just get started!

Once you have measured your HuDGE, the next obvious question would be how to improve your HuDGE? How to build a strong HuDGE? Let's find out in the next chapter.

HuDGE	
Components	**Elements**
1. Continuity	1. How many families rely on you as single point of contact
	2. What is the follow-up rate or attrition rate of your patients and how good is their compliance or monitoring?
	3. How many doctors are there in your referral network? How many patients you refer and how many you get as referrals?
2. Clinical Outcomes	1. How well are you able to longitudinally track health status of your patients?
	2. How many Emergency Room admissions were avoided?
	3. In case in-patient care was required, were you in loop during admission and after discharge?
4. Word of Mouth	1. In what proportion of your patients do you involve their families in providing care and educate them?
	2. How many of the new families who got associated with you were referred by your existing patients and their families?
	3. What proportion of your patients or their families know about your achievements from time to time?

Table 2: What's your HuDGE?

CHAPTER 7

The HuDGE Playbook: How to Improve Your HuDGE?

"If you can't explain it simply, you don't understand it well enough"

– Albert Einstein

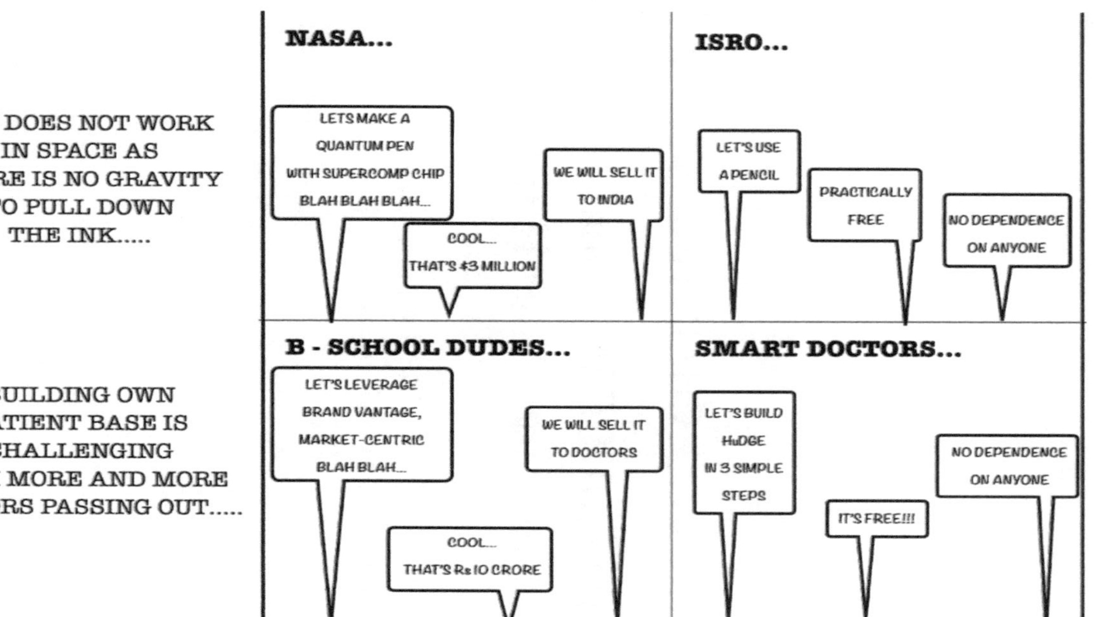
PEN DOES NOT WORK
IN SPACE AS
THERE IS NO GRAVITY
TO PULL DOWN
THE INK.....
NASA...
LETS MAKE A
QUANTUM PEN
WITH SUPERCOMP CHIP
BLAH BLAH BLAH...
COOL...
THAT'S $3 MILLION
WE WILL SELL IT
TO INDIA
ISRO...
LET'S USE
A PENCIL
PRACTICALLY
FREE
NO DEPENDENCE
ON ANYONE
BUILDING OWN
PATIENT BASE IS
CHALLENGING
WITH MORE AND MORE
DOCTORS PASSING OUT.....
B - SCHOOL DUDES...
LET'S LEVERAGE
BRAND VANTAGE,
MARKET-CENTRIC
BLAH BLAH...
COOL...
THAT'S Rs 10 CRORE
WE WILL SELL IT
TO DOCTORS
SMART DOCTORS...
LET'S BUILD
HuDGE
IN 3 SIMPLE
STEPS
IT'S FREE!!!
NO DEPENDENCE
ON ANYONE

Once you have measured your HuDGE and identified areas of improvement, the next step is to improve your HuDGE. Perhaps this is what you were looking forward to when you started reading this book. As Albert Einstein rightly said "If you can't explain it simply, you don't understand it well enough". In order to keep it simple, easy to understand and easy to implement, we have distilled different facets from our research. Behold, you just need to do three things to strengthen your HuDGE. Yes, you read it right just three things!

First, build "My patient treasury"

My patient treasury is where you add all your patients and record all consultations you give on a daily basis. Start recording/ counting-in all the consultations you give, even the informal opinions or off-hand consultations that you would invariably be giving to your relatives, families, neighbors and friends. Are we suggesting you should put a price tag on each one of them? DEFINITELY NOT! That is purely your purview. Most of you do it for free on a goodwill and you can continue doing the same, just that you need to record them and channelize these consults in a systematic fashion.

That way you can have a track of your progress and your patients will also take it more seriously. Adding every patient to my patient treasury and giving all consultations through it, even when giving free off-hand informal consults, will give you an idea about how big is your patient base and also can show you how fast it is growing with time. You will find this data extremely helpful when you are planning to invest in setting up your own clinic. You would know where and when to invest without losing money. You could also possibly use this while negotiating with private hospitals or corporate chains because patient base is one thing no one can ignore.

As we have elaborated in the previous chapters, you need to start by being single point of contact (SPOC) for not just patients but their families as well. So, when do you start? Early bird gets the worm, so now is a good time. I would say you can start on the same day you register your MBBS with the medical council. If you are a MBBS graduate and studying for NEET and other PG entrance exams, it's a good time to start. If you are a PG resident doctor or Registrar doing your MD/MS/DNB it's definitely a good time to start. If you are doing your Senior Residency or working as a Junior Consultant or planning to start your own private practice, well it is high time you start!

Where can you start? Charity begins at home. You can start with your family, relatives, neighbors, friends and their extended families. Many of you during your PG entrance exam preparation would be working part time (we have all been through that!). This can be a good start for "My Patient Treasury".

When you enter PG or super specialty residency programmes like MD/MS/DM/MCH or DNB, you would invariably slog round-the-clock. You will be seeing numerous patients in OPD, hospital corridors, canteens and even outside restaurants (when they get to know you are a doctor!). Imagine if you could start building "My patient treasury" right from this time. You will have a ready patient base by the time you come out as a specialist or a super specialist.

I have known some of my seniors during PG residency program who would diligently give their WhatsApp numbers to all their patients and ensured continuity. Obviously, they did not waste a single day after their MD and straightaway started their own clinics. Opening a clinic involves cost and they could confidently do it only because they had a ready patience base. Few other seniors smartly negotiated favorable financial contracts with private/Corporate hospitals citing their existing patient base. So, when you see some of your own seniors and friends establishing themselves earlier than the others, take a closer look, they would definitely have started building their patient base much before the others.

Second, build "My referral network"

Medical science is expanding rapidly by the day. As practicing doctors, we invariably refer patients to our fellow doctors from different specialties and vice versa. Therefore, referrals are an extremely important part in your clinical practice. In fact, your importance and position also heavily depends on it. As most of you would have noticed only a few Cardiologists, Neurologists, Surgeons among others, actually become star consultants. The hard truth is that a significant chunk of superspecialists are struggling to establish themselves.

In fact, the more a doctor specializes, the more she/ he would be dependent on referrals for the simple reason that they would be focusing only on niche areas and therefore patients do not directly go to them. On the other hand, many general practitioners are in a commanding position because they are the first point of contact for patients and consequently act as gateway for referrals. They would have established themselves in specific localities and hold a vantage point in terms of patient base.

Patients very well understand that their doctors are not experts in everything and they appreciate it when you are candid enough to tell them the same. From your patients' point of view, they feel reassured knowing that you can get them across to the right specialist as and when required. It is always better to refer a patient to your colleague within your referral network because the patient eventually comes back to you. This helps to maintain continuity of care and also retain your patient base.

Besides, as the saying goes "*Nothing is free and not all prices appear on labels*". Your value amongst your peers would depend on how many referrals you can potentially make and vice versa. To be professionally successful you need a good network of fellow doctors. Systematically building "My referral network" can help you actually identify the right set of colleagues who can be a part of your network. A weak referral network is one of the common causes for loss to follow-up and break in continuity of care. "My referral network" can address this and also helps to retain your patients within your network.

So, when is the right time to start? It's now. From where do you start? If you are a MBBS graduate preparing for PG entrance exams, you would anyways be giving many informal, off-hand consultations. You would invariably be referring one in three patients that you see to some of your own seniors who are specialists. It is a good opportunity to add your seniors to your referral network and retain your patient base. The same is the case if you are a PG student or doing your senior residency.

If you are planning to start your practice, you should definitely add your juniors who have recently graduated and other GPs (General Practitioners) to your referral network. As you move up the specialization ladder, it is only your referral network that will help you to get established. An unsaid rule is, to get referrals you should also have sent referrals and therefore building your referral network early-on in your career definitely gives you an edge.

In the process, you also need to phase-out any form of intermediaries. It is a good idea to anonymize service providers like pharmacy, labs etc who interact with patients to minimize the chances of patients being misled. Needless to say, it is better to keep away from aggregators as they are likely to divert your patients for commissions due to their very business model, as discussed in the previous chapter.

Third, "Quantify and Showcase your impact"

The third thing you need to do is quantify your impact! Let's understand this. One of the common grouses and perception people have about private practitioners and private sector is perceived over treatment. There is a growing perception that the current healthcare system is trying to push people into hospitals. This by the way is partly true, considering the very business models and market forces that are operating (Refer chapter 3). Of late, the focus is predominantly on the illness side of the spectrum with little or no time given to the wellness side. This trend has only added to the vicious cycle of growing trust deficit.

Therefore, it is extremely important for us as doctors to start focusing on the wellness aspects along with managing the illnesses. It is equally important that the patients and their families know and perceive that you are more wellness centric and *doing your best to keep them out of hospitals*. As discussed in the previous chapters, by virtue of information asymmetry and high perceived risk of a wrong decision, doctors are in a position to nudge patients to make the right choices all along. Right from the stage of preventing diseases to early diagnosis, compliance to treatment, choosing a hospital, prevention of complications and rehabilitation, patients' choices are heavily influenced by their doctors. This is essentially the Human Nudge aka HuDGE, where doctor is the human capable of creating a Nudge. As you start and continue your HuDGE, it reinforces the trust and makes it easier to further HuDGE and your patients will be your brand ambassadors in the community.

Okay that's pretty theoretical. How do we actually do this? Well, the broad principle is you try to keep your patients out of hospitals. In case they need in-patient care, help them choose the specialist and hospital for their condition. Once they get admitted work with the admitting physician, stay updated about patient condition and try to minimize the hospital stay. Get the patient back to full functionality post-discharge at the earliest. HuDGE involves systematically using appropriate tools at each of these stages to measure and demonstrate improvements. Being able to see improvements motivates patients and also shows your patients how much your presence is actually helping them.

HuDGE your patients with disease specific risk assessment tools. It can be a good start. Not just you, your patients also get to know their health risk. Then HuDGE them to adopt preventive measures specific to their disease conditions. This would require customized suggestions for every patient. This can be done by recognizing patterns pertaining to their demographic details, family history, lifestyle choices and overall compliance. As Medicos, we are all trained to connect these dots in every patient we see. We just need to systematically carry this out wherein the patient and their families can also be a part of it and see the improvements.

Imagine the difference it would make when you show your patients what is the probability that he might get admitted in the next one year with complications. Think of the wow factor when your patient is told how many times his Emergency Room admissions were prevented because of you. The happiness your patients would have just to know you were actively following up their condition while in hospital and facilitated timely discharge. The satisfaction your patients will have knowing how many days they saved in getting back to normalcy because of you.

This requires use of scientifically validated specialty and disease specific tools. Then you need customized

HuDGE clinical programmes for each of your patients. Not all patients are same nor are their disease conditions. There will surely be some early adopters. You need to first work closely with them, bring out results and portray them as examples to the late adopters and laggards. There will always be a small fraction of non-compliant, non-adopters. Nonetheless, with a systematic approach you can HuDGE more than 90% of your patients.

Human mind works best on contrast and comparisons. HuDGE your patients with objective evidence/ information on your impact as their doctor and you can be sure of stronger continuity, better clinical outcomes and assured word of mouth popularity.

Alright, so can you do this all by yourself? Of course, YES. In fact, if you see any successful practitioner, they will be good at all three things or doing at least one of them very well. Generally, GPs are good at "My patient treasury". They are good at building patient base. Successful super-specialists will invariably have a very strong referral network. Successful specialists dealing with chronic diseases like Diabetes Mellitus, Hypertension, Chronic Kidney Disease, psychiatric illnesses etc would be good at quantifying their impact.

They are all doing it manually and it is working just fine. Just that it can get laborious and time consuming when done manually apart from missing out on details when workload increases. You can save a lot of time and effort by doing the same things systematically using appropriate technology, the HuDGE technology. Scan the QR code in Chapter 12 and use your unique access code to get started.

CHAPTER 8

The Corporate Constantinople: Why Should the Corporates Care?

"If you don't learn from history, you are
doomed to repeat it."

– George Santayana.

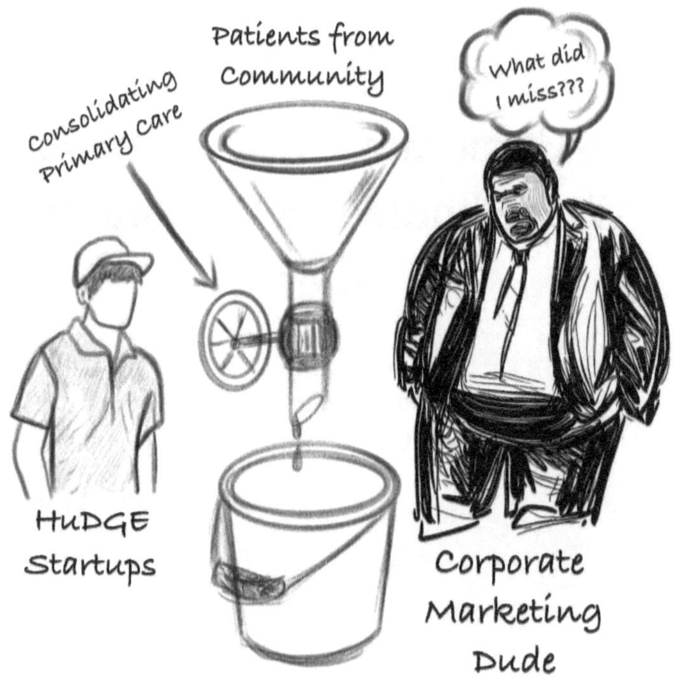
Consolidating Primary Care
Patients from Community
What did I miss???
HuDGE Startups
Corporate Marketing Dude

Corporate hospital chains have contributed immensely to the development of Indian healthcare over the last few decades. They have played a vital role in bringing world-class technology to India at a time when patients had to go abroad for advanced therapies. This not only delayed treatment but also created huge inequities as mostly the rich could afford going abroad. They filled a vital gap in Indian healthcare at a time when the government was struggling to pitch in.

The corporates have pioneered the concepts of continuous quality improvement, quality accreditation, patient safety, clinical excellence among others, all of which are patient-centric. They have mastered the art of providing the best-in-class treatment at a fraction of the cost compared to the US or Europe. Their financial prowess of negotiating the best prices based on large volumes has unequivocally benefited the common man. Just to give a perspective knee replacement that costs $17,500 in the US is done at $6,600 dollars in India, an angioplasty costs $5,700 in India compared to $17,700 in the US and IVF costs $2,500 in India vis a vis $14,900 in the US [1]. Treatment cost in the US is about three to six times more expensive than India. Thanks to the relentless efforts of our visionary healthcare leaders, Indian healthcare is standing up to the global standards and is on the world map as one of the leading destinations for medical value tourism a.k.a. medical tourism.

Everything seems upbeat and sunny right? What is the problem? Well, there's another side. Despite heavy investments and efforts, corporate chains are struggling to establish themselves in smaller cities and towns. Their presence is largely in the metro cities and to some extent in tier 1 cities which have now turned into red oceans with many new players coming in.

Report of Sub-Group-IV of Expert Committee on Enhancing Resource Investment in Health (ECERIH) commissioned by the Government of India states that Corporate Hospitals account for just around 1% of total hospitals in India and 67% of corporate hospitals are clustered in just 8 big Indian cities [2]. It would be interesting to know that more than 80% of hospitals in India are less than 50 bedded "mom and pops" facilities [3]. Healthcare in India continues to be strongly hyperlocal.

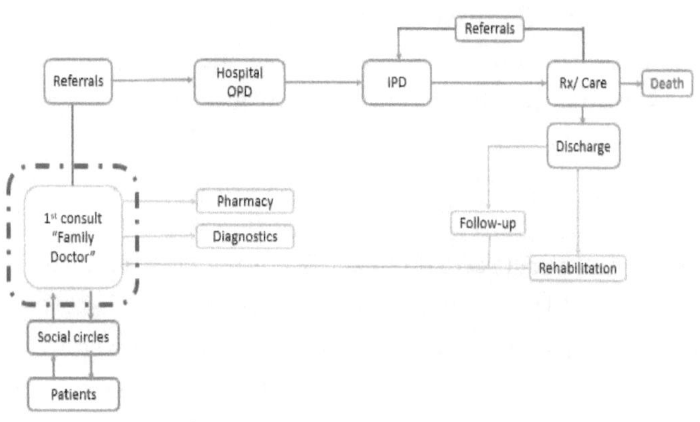

Figure 1: Healthcare Value Chain in India

Let's try and understand this better through the healthcare value chain in India. When we study the general behavior among majority of patients, their journey often starts with their trusted social circles which is invariably followed by their trusted doctor in close vicinity. For our discussion, Let's call her/him "Family Doctor". The subsequent decisions of undergoing investigations, taking medications or for that matter, going to a bigger hospital for secondary or tertiary care are strongly influenced by their respective family doctors. These doctors are the single point of contact for their patients.

Irrespective of their specialty or degrees, they are the first port of call for any healthcare related queries of their patients. The patients also come back and double check advice received from other specialists with their "Family Doctors". They are the guardians who strongly influence and practically control the gateway to secondary and tertiary healthcare. The journey of the patients through the remaining parts of healthcare value chain including patients' choice of hospital depends on these Family Doctors.

That boils down to a deceptively simple and a touchy question of whether the patients come in the name of their doctors or just by the name/ glamour of corporate chains? We all understand the power of branding. However, we also know that value of a brand cannot be quantified and it is difficult to measure the real impact of any form of conventional ATL or BTL marketing. We have seen how these conventional marketing approaches, digital marketing, social media and aggregators fall flat when it comes to healthcare, despite having worked extremely well for other sectors like FMCG, finance, entertainment etc.

Simply put, being a pioneer or market leader in certain types of high-end procedures or technology and widely publicizing it may give an edge over competitor brands. But when we ask ourselves, what can influence patients' decision more? A large billboard or Frontpage newspaper ad versus suggestion by their Family Doctor? The answer is pretty clear. The family doctor's suggestion almost always supersedes any other form of marketing influences. We have discussed and understood different factors responsible for this like information asymmetry, hyperlocal markets, social capital and cultural aspects in the previous chapters.

When organizations start to expand and scale, it is common to see that processes take precedence over people. Increase in size and complexities creates bureaucratization and the organizations tend to become more "impersonal". Customers can increasingly feel they are dealing with a faceless albeit sophisticated system rather than an empathetic person who really cares about them. This trend can be especially damaging for healthcare organizations who may end up in the Corporate Chakravyuha.

This starts with lack of personal connect with people in the community. This makes it increasingly difficult and therefore more expensive to bring in patients prompting "marketing for the sake of marketing" with heavy expenditure on ATL and BTL. These culminate in higher customer acquisition cost (CAC) and other overheads. This can further increase the cost of care/treatment which in turn increases the trust gap and makes personal connect more difficult to achieve.

Increasing competition with newer corporate chains operating in the same urban pockets only aggravates this vicious cycle. We can correlate with the Nash equilibrium of game theory. New players backed by investments tend to spend heavily on marketing activities. They are merely mimicking the customer acquisition process of FMCGs where a new brand adopts a bullish aggressive marketing campaign to make its presence felt. This invariably intimidates and prompts the incumbent players also to up the ante and spend more on their marketing.

The "marketing dudes" are undoubtedly brilliant in selling toothpaste and sugar water. But it is just not the same in healthcare and all their assumptions fall flat. They apply the same principles of enhancing consumption to increase volumes and are nowhere close to HuDGE, setting in a vicious cycle of corporate Chakravyuha.

Coming back to the healthcare value chain, we understand the power of family doctors in the whole scheme of things. Currently almost the entire primary health care in India is provided by unorganized or informal sector. They are strongly hyper local which means even if an entity manages to substitute the family doctor in one part of a city by using some exotic innovative strategy, it will not be able to use the same strategy even in the neighboring locality. This makes it practically impossible for any entity or company to consolidate or acquire this critical part of the health care value chain.

For easy understanding of my medico friends let's try to understand the meaning of scalability using a simple comparison with toothpaste. Let's say there is a new company which wants to sell toothpaste. They would first identify their target segment, say for example college going kids. They would then prepare a list of things that any usual college kid would aspire for. They then narrow down on one theme that would appeal to any college going kid, say "the fear of losing friends due to bad breath". Next, they design a marketing campaign to convince people that they could actually have a problem of bad breath and use fear or paranoia to subconsciously reinforce this thought. In the same flow they portray their new toothpaste as the only solution for this problem of bad breath. Now they continuously bombard people with these ads on billboards newspaper ads, ads during IPL, you name it. At every corner, in every conversation, they are just trying to flood you. Have you noticed something very interesting about this? Right from Kashmir to Kanyakumari, from Metro cities to remote villages, from hills to plain areas, from desert to evergreen forests, these marketing campaigns remain the same except for adaptation in regional languages. Now, this my friends is called scalability. Once you know, certain type of marketing has worked in a pilot run in some areas you can almost certainly expect it to work across the length and breadth of the country. Some are trying to replicate this approach in healthcare through ATL and BTL. But the very nature of Indian healthcare being hyper local does not make it amenable to these conventional approaches. Now we know why blindly copy-pasting marketing from other industries is not a good idea.

Now let us imagine that HuDGE is systematized and made mainstream by an insignificant inconspicuous start-up. Let us say this start-up empowers every single doctor to measure and strengthen her/ his HuDGE and works towards strengthening doctor patient relationship. It helps the doctors be independent entrepreneurs that they always wanted to be. Now that is the *Corporate Constantinople!*

By the way, most of us would be wondering what is Constantinople? For my medico friends, long story short, today's Istanbul in Turkey was previously called Constantinople. Being the link between Europe and Asia the city was the Gateway for trade between the two continents and two seas (the Mediterranean and the Black Sea). Due to its strategic location, the city practically controlled the trade between Europe and Asia.

It had enormous riches which is even today evident from beautiful buildings like Hagia Sophia, The Imperial Palace, the Golden Gate among many others. Consequently, it was also a centre for art and literature. It served as the capital for byzantine Roman Empire. It was known for its fortification which prevented external invasions for almost 900 years.

However, it came under repeated attacks from the Arabs and the city finally fell in the year 1453 which historians call *Fall of Constantinople*. This was a watershed moment in the history of commerce, trade and largely mankind. The Arabs started levying heavy taxes on all forms of trade going through Constantinople. The traders in the Europe were practically cut off from Asian supplies of spices, silk Gold and all other goods.

Now if we draw a parallel with the healthcare value chain in India, we can consider the layer of family doctors as equivalent to the historic Constantinople. The family doctors are practically the Gateway for patients to the rest of Indian healthcare, just like Constantinople was the gateway for Europe to entire Asia. Constantinople was famous for its massive and complex fortifications, which ranked among the most sophisticated defensive architecture of antiquity. The Theodosian walls with the intricate topography made it difficult for the external powers to break through or even understand it. Likewise, the Indian family doctors are hyperlocal, from different walks of life, have different qualifications and belong to varied specialties. These intricate features along with patient behavior influenced by cultural aspects have always remained an enigma. This is possibly why no corporate entity has been able to consolidate or control it.

Even the tech giants like Google and Microsoft have tried, failed and still wondering what they are missing in healthcare. Considering the amount of financial and intellectual capital they own; we should be happy they haven't got a hang of this yet. None of them have been able to penetrate the Indian family doctors. Clearly, it takes way more than just pumping money and building software.

Now let's say the insignificant inconspicuous start-ups we just mentioned manage to reach the Indian family doctors. They would have practically gotten the Constantinople of Indian healthcare!!! The corporate chains would gradually but surely have to depend on them to get referrals and patients. This will send their customer acquisition cost over the roof. Basically, it would cost the corporates way more money to get the patients up to the hospitals. The situation could be similar to that of the Medieval period European traders who faced existential crisis as it only got harder to access the Asian markets when Constantinople fell to the Ottoman Empire. *That is what we call the corporate Constantinople!!!*

History is bereft with many such examples wherein some cornerstone events have changed the course of industries. Motorola produced one of the best pagers and was the undisputed market leader. However, they didn't see the smartphones coming. They lost most of the ground and their phones continue to struggle even till date. Likewise, Microsoft was slow to catch up with the smartphone revolution and is now paying Google to allow its browsers. Google led the smartphone revolution and quickly acquired Customers/users around the world. Majority of them have leapfrogged desktops and started with smartphones.

Apple's app tracking policy has been the tech world's one of the recent linchpins. If you are an iPhone user you would have noticed that when you download or open any app, the phone gives you an option to refuse permission to that app to track your activities across different apps. Ever wondered how the same things that you search on Google starts appearing on your Facebook or Instagram page? Well, that is because the apps that we use track our activity and data across all other apps.

This helps the tech companies to understand our needs, profile us and show customized advertisements which increases the chances of buying. Apple's recent app tracking policy has dealt a death blow to Facebook and Google since it is now harder for them to track our activities across other apps. The commonality in all these examples is, one windfall event in the gateways controlling or influencing consumers behavior, can make or break empires and companies alike.

The real threat for luxury car manufacturers like Mercedes is not Audi or Jaguar. The real threat is from the mutual funds. Mutual funds promote the behavior of savings and therefore deters the neo-rich or upper middle class from splurging on luxury goods. Its impact in India has been significant enough for Mercedes to reportedly issue a "SIP warning".

In this context, *the real threat to any corporate hospital chain is not a competing corporate entity. The real threat is any innovation that can consolidate the Indian Family Doctors who are the Gateway to secondary and tertiary healthcare.* Any external shock waves or windfall events can potentially jeopardize their financial health which was also seen during COVID-19 pandemic.

So, what can the corporates do? A new trend of "increasing presence in primary care" is coming up. Some corporate chains have started opening clinics which are expected to function as feeder channels or outpatient funnels for the hospital business. Merely increasing the points of care or infrastructure doesn't help much. With time these clinics add up to the financial overheads if they cannot build and strengthen HuDGE.

Corporates need to leverage their strengths in building tech that patients in the community can use. A project like the Smart-Colpo can be a good "loss leader" for corporate chains especially the ones dealing with oncology [4]. They will have to build their own HuDGE clinical programs through strong "Tech engagement" of both doctors and patients. We should stop spilling the beans and let the "marketing dudes" do some thinking. Let's move on.

CHAPTER 9

End of the Road for Health Care Aggregators?

"Culture eats strategy for breakfast"

– Peter Druker

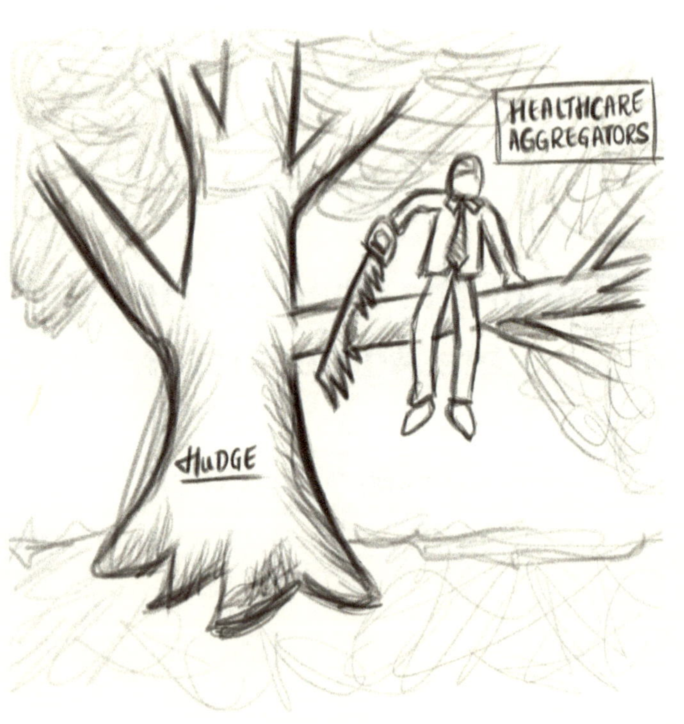

HEALTHCARE
AGGREGATORS
HUDGE

There has been a growing discontent among doctors about aggregators who are involved in diverting their patients for higher commissions. The honorable Delhi High Court has sought an explanation regarding a petition against health service aggregators over allegedly misleading advertisements, ridiculous discounts and unsolicited messages[1]. There are also grouses about unethical selling practices adopted by some of them. Many of these aggregators have also been in news of late for laying off many employees citing financial constraints and decreasing business. So, what exactly is happening? Aggregators are many times portrayed as "Unicorns" with many high-profile examples from other domains. Then why are the healthcare aggregators struggling?

To understand this better, let's get down to the basics. Aggregators basically work on an e-commerce model. This further can be either a marketplace model where the aggregator provides only the platform for buyers and sellers or could be an inventory model wherein the aggregator themselves hold or store the items that they sell online. Okay, let's not complicate it. In short aggregators spend lots of money on digital marketing and deep discounts to attract more online buyers. They also bring in sellers on board, assuring them of certain minimum business. They use these volumes or large number of buyers to negotiate cheaper prices from the sellers and the cycle continues.

The idea behind any e-commerce venture is to eliminate the middlemen or intermediaries. They practically remove the human interface and connects the buyers directly to the sellers. This has turned out to be a revolutionary concept as it brings in more efficiency ease and transparency for both buyers and sellers. It has also empowered many small businesses and micro-Entrepreneurs who can now sell their products to any customer across the length and Breadth of the country without having to depend on local distributors, supermarkets or shopkeepers. This model has created unicorns after unicorns in consumer goods, electronics, fashion commodities, clothing, groceries, insurance, banking, finance, cab services, transports, education, food & beverages and many more. You name it, you will find some or the other aggregator in almost every commodity or service that you require on a daily basis. A whole lot of them have been a raging success as well. They have undoubtedly been visionaries who have scripted history with their contribution and success. They have set a new benchmark for entrepreneurship and shown that anything is achievable. So far so good?

Okay now let's look at some interesting data. We all know of Amazon, one of the largest e-commerce platforms. If we go by the stats put up on Shiprocket site, Amazon has more than 10 Crore registered users in India and sells more than 4000 products every minute and yet Amazon is struggling to decrease its losses. According to a survey data, 82% of people who buy online reported that they buy online because of big discounts [2]. Amazon e-commerce marketplace is still not profitable, Amazon Web services and Amazon prime are actually the cash cows for Amazon. Flipkart being one of the largest e-commerce platforms has also reported losses.

So how do they actually make money and sustain? That's an entirely different topic of discussion. In the interest of simplicity, let's say they are floating with investors' money and have a high valuation because of their user base. The valuation is based on the premise that once a user visits a platform, the platforms can sell other items to these users and multiply their revenue. The general trend is that there is an initial phase of cash burn where many of the aggregators spend heavily to acquire customers and retain them. With time, the aggregators figure out newer monetization strategies (just a jargon for ways of making more money) from the users they have acquired. This is followed by a point of breakeven wherein their revenues start increasing and cash burn to acquire customers starts decreasing. When this continues for long enough, these companies can become profitable. It would be interesting to note that many of these start-ups are still in the cash burn phase and are yet to become profitable.

Some visionary entrepreneurs have tried to build aggregators in healthcare on similar e-commerce business models. They have replaced the consumers with patients and have placed doctors as sellers. This is an awesome business model, right? Where is the problem?

According to an editorial in Invest India, e-pharmacies have been around for close to a decade with around 50 e-pharmacies currently operating and yet they have managed just around 2-3% of the total Indian pharmacy sales. Traditional pharma retail in India is highly unorganized and fragmented with close to 8.5 lakh unorganized retailers contributing more than 90% of sales[3]. Clearly the e-pharmacies have not been able to stand up to the local pharmacy shops.

On the other hand, some of the successful fashion aggregators, restaurant aggregators (food delivery apps), cab aggregators have been around for almost the same time but have been seemingly more successful in terms of building their user base by reaching out to more and more people. If we consider number of users acquired as a measure of success, then fin tech companies like Google pay, PhonePe, BharatPe etc have been far more successful in probably just half the time.

The common justification is that fin-tech companies got a massive tailwind from demonetization and UPI infrastructure. From that perspective, healthcare aggregators and health tech companies also got tailwind of the century, the COVID-19 pandemic. Right from e-pharmacies, home diagnostics to tele-health, all of them saw tremendous growth during the pandemic. But as the fear of the pandemic started weaning off, these companies started losing business. The recent massive lay-offs by some of the leading health-tech companies and healthcare aggregators citing poor market conditions clearly reflects that they could not sustain the momentary growth and opportunity provided by the pandemic. This is in contrast to the fin-tech companies which took off during demonetization and have continued to rapidly grow ever since by adding more and more users with time.

What went wrong? What are the healthcare aggregators missing? We should always remember that it is easier to connect the dots looking backwards. It is easier to criticize policies sitting on armchair and this is my favorite, it is easier to say Dhoni or Kohli should have played an off-drive instead of a straight drive. We should salute the Spirit of entrepreneurship. The idea is not to criticize but to critically analyze, to improve and move forward. Let's try and understand why a model that has worked extremely well for other sectors may not be the best fit for health care.

First, it is the consumer profile. Majority of people who need healthcare are in their late 40s and 50s. Just about 10% of people in India speak English and most of them are not tech savvy. Barely 2-3% of Indian population is currently availing healthcare services through smart-phones. Besides, information asymmetry is a real challenge as discussed in the previous chapters.

The second aspect is Consumer engagement. How frequently and how well the users engage with the apps determines their user retention. Nir Eyal in his book "Hooked" beautifully explains the four stages of the hook cycle. Let us say you want to order food, book a cab or buy groceries, you will subconsciously open the app that you are "accustomed to". In cases of such apps that are used on a daily basis; billboards, front page newspaper ads, sponsored ads on Google search adds to their brand recognition and brand recall.

Now let's take healthcare apps. Patients with chronic illnesses like diabetes, hypertension, chronic kidney disease etc mostly require a consult once in a few months. They generally require medication refill once in a couple of months. So technically patients with known illnesses themselves would think of the app at most once in a couple of months. There are no factors to get the patients "accustomed to" these apps. These apps are just not sticky enough! Therefore, by the next time if their neighborhood pharmacy or Lab offers them the same convenience, the patients are more likely to choose them.

Some of these aggregators try cold calls which are known to have very low success rate and are especially irritating. Many of them try bulk SMS campaigns which again have doubtful efficacy. A cold SMS for someone who doesn't have the need to get a consult, buy medicines or get blood test can at the most create irritation. In the absence of "Tech tie-in" consumers engagement in most of the healthcare apps is low and no amount of conventional or digital marketing can replace it.

The third is Cultural aspects. The very cultural fabric in India and the ways in which social capital functions make healthcare largely driven by trust, personal contacts and word of mouth. These cultural factors are so strong that healthcare remains predominantly hyper-local despite heavy investments and efforts, to turn it the other way round. Health tech companies and aggregators despite having the best in class, cutting-edge technology are mostly faceless, impersonal interfaces. They are missing the Human Nudge/ HuDGE and are trying to swim against the very culture that can eat their strategy for breakfast.

The very design of e-commerce models do not encourage continuity with the same doctor/ provider. This naturally has a cascading effect on clinical outcomes which by the way are seldom measured by the incumbent players. So, this naturally rules out any form of word of mouth. In summary, the health tech companies or aggregators do not fulfil any of the three components or 9 elements of HuDGE which could be the main reason for their current situation.

CHAPTER 10

Start-ups; What Should They Do?

"The next Bill Gates will not make an Operating System; the next Larry Page will not make a search engine and the next Zuckerberg will not make a social networking site"

– Peter Thiel

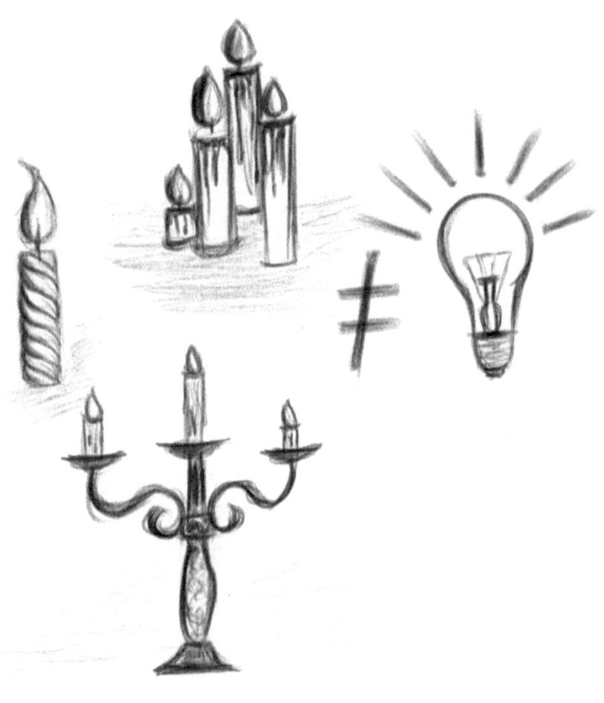

We are neither motivational speakers nor self-proclaimed gurus who gives punchlines and stories. We will not tell you any fancy rags to riches stories of unicorns or their founders. Though we should certainly celebrate their success as ours. We will just stick to facts and figures and what needs to be done. So, this is going to be the shortest chapter in the book.

This is the best time to be a start-up in India. In 2021 we added a unicorn every 29 days, in 2022 we added a unicorn every 9 days[1]. There are numerous factors that decide or influence the success of a start-up. But the most important among them is getting the right problem statement. Unless you are solving a relevant problem, that really means something to your users, you cannot get far.

Dr. Devi Shetty during one of his talks at AIIMS New Delhi said that "The next big thing in healthcare will not be a hospital or a group of hospitals, but a piece of technology" while pointing towards his phone. Throughout this book, we have understood the importance of the Human Nudge aka HuDGE in healthcare. We have also seen how merely replicating the business models from other sectors may not yield the desired results. A successful product is the one which can acquire customers at low-cost, engage them by understanding consumers behavior, retain them by solving their problems and monetize the users in a way that users also see value in it.

As for customer acquisition, unless you are backed by your father (or father-in-law!) with tons of cash to spare, the usual approach of customer acquisition through a big ticket ATL/BTL or Digital marketing may not be a sustainable option for healthcare start-ups. Customer engagement and retention can become a nightmare as people remember of healthcare services once in a few months, mostly during distress. Therefore, just building an app and expecting the patients will automatically start using it by themselves is not a wise thing to do. This approach will definitely not work, even if the app is sophisticated and technologically advanced. The natural consequence is you will not be able to optimally monetize your user base and end up with cash burn.

Peter Thiel, co-founder of PayPal, rightly says that "The next Bill Gates will not build an Operating System, the next Larry Page won't build a search engine and the next Mark Zukerberg won't build a social network. If you are copying from these guys, you aren't learning from them". Simply copying an existing model from some other sector is easy to do, but is unlikely to fetch much.

So how to go about? Well, the three components and nine elements of HuDGE provides an excellent reference point. Whenever you are building a product, just see if it fits into any of the nine elements of HuDGE. The more elements you touch upon and address, the better would be your chances of success. If you are a medico and up for it, we are here to support you.

We should stop here and let the founders kindle their brains!!!

CHAPTER 11

What Will the Future Look Like?

"The Light bulb did not come by continuous improvement of candles"

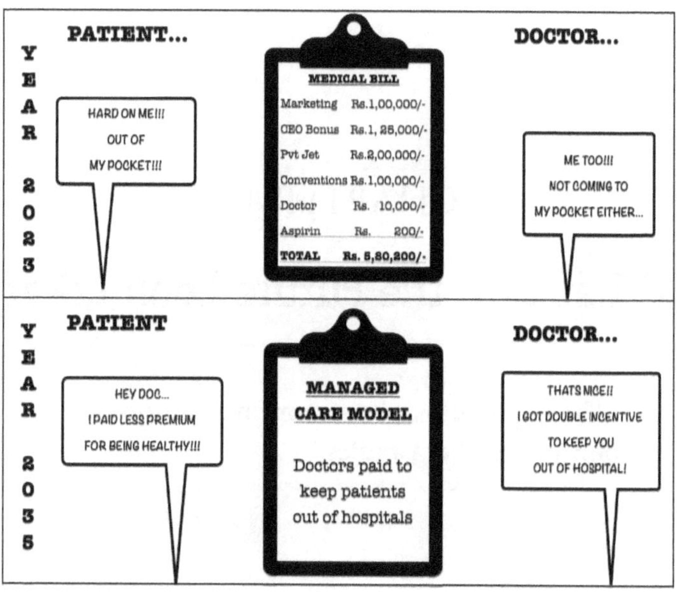
YEAR 2023
PATIENT...
HARD ON ME!!!
OUT OF
MY POCKET!!!
MEDICAL BILL
Marketing Rs.1,00,000/-
CEO Bonus Rs.1, 25,000/-
Pvt Jet Rs.2,00,000/-
Conventions Rs.1,00,000/-
Doctor Rs. 10,000/-
Aspirin Rs. 200/-
TOTAL Rs. 5,80,200/-
DOCTOR...
ME TOO!!!
NOT COMING TO
MY POCKET EITHER...
YEAR 2035
PATIENT
HEY DOC...
I PAID LESS PREMIUM
FOR BEING HEALTHY!!!
MANAGED CARE MODEL
Doctors paid to keep patients out of hospitals
DOCTOR...
THATS NICE!!
I GOT DOUBLE INCENTIVE
TO KEEP YOU
OUT OF HOSPITAL!

Just in the last 20 years or so, Indian health care has seen paradigm shifts. There have been many cornerstone events which at the time did not seem very important but have actually contributed immensely to the changes. The National Rural Health Mission (NRHM) was launched in 2005 and created grassroot level healthcare workers like ASHA, Anganwadi workers, ANMs. etc. It has created tectonic shifts in our health indicators despite some shortcomings. There have been definite improvements in our IMR (Infant Mortality Rates), MMR, Vaccination cover for children, Under five mortality and others. Many of these initiatives could control communicable diseases so much so that noncommunicable diseases now account for almost 60% of deaths. This can also be seen as people are living long enough to develop noncommunicable diseases like hypertension, diabetes, cancers, etc which are now the leading cause of death.

There have been various state sponsored insurance schemes like RSBY, Aarogyashree etc which over the years were envisioned to cater to the poor and underprivileged. With all these learnings came Ayushmann Bharat-Pradhan Mantri Jan Arogya Yojana (AB-PMJAY), the world's largest government funded health insurance programme that covers almost 10 Crore families or 50 crore individuals. Then came COVID-19 pandemic which turned the system upside down and created an existential threat to many players in the industry.

Historically, it is evident that any major change be it a precipitous revolution or an insidious evolution, has happened due to changes in flow of money or information. This is possibly because information, authentic or otherwise, can mold opinions and thought process. Money provides the necessary means to convert these thoughts into actions. Be it the outcome of the second world war or the world order after it, change in flow of information and money have always played an important role. Part of the reason for the dominating position of the US is the US dollar being the de facto currency for majority of international trade and commerce. Likewise, if not for the LPG reforms in India in the 1990s, which eased the flow of money coming into and going out of India, we would probably still be waiting for months at length for a landline, scooter, car or even cooking gas connection at the mercy of some government run *"Sarkaari"* companies. The IT industry boom was both an outcome and a catalyst in changing the flow of information and money. If not for this, we would probably not have the kind of economic growth and employment that we see today.

Demonetization and UPI are a landmark example of how change in flow of money and information can practically create a whole new sector of digital payments and fin-tech. India now has more than 2300 UPI transactions every second[1]. It took India 67 years to become a $1 trillion economy. It took another 8 years to reach the $2 trillion Mark and thanks to UPI and digital payments, we have reached $3 trillion mark in just 5 years[2].

Now let's understand how changes in flow of money and information will impact healthcare. This can equip us to be better prepared for the changes. Let's start with the change in flow of money. AB-PMJAY has been envisioned as the largest government funded health insurance programme that covers about 10 Crore families and 50 Crore individuals. This landmark scheme is aimed at providing essential health care cover to the poor and underprivileged. The recent report by NITI Aayog on the missing Middle highlights that approximately 30 Crore Indians still do not have any form of health insurance cover. They are the middle class who are not poor enough to be covered by government schemes and not rich enough to afford buying private health insurance covers [3]. The insurance cover has dramatically increased over the years. So how does this even matter to us as practicing doctors and how can it change the industry?

Currently almost 100% of outpatient services are out-of-pocket expenditure for patients. With increasing penetration of insurance, government of India has managed to save close to Rs. 1 Lakh Crore expenditure that patient would have otherwise paid out of their pockets [4]. As the insurance penetration increases, the flow of money is bound to change. Right now, patients pay out of pocket. But with insurance coverage, insurance companies become their payors.

For any insurance company to sustain they predominantly need three things. First, is risk pooling. This means they need large number of subscribers whose premiums is the major source of revenue. Second, they need risk estimation or actuaries as they are called. As many of us would know, the health insurance premium increases with age, comorbid medical conditions, any past history of illnesses and so on. That way, the insurance company knows the probability of any of its subscribers falling ill. The more the risk of falling ill, the more will be the premium. Third they need risk mitigation. This simply means that the insurance companies make more profit when more and more of their subscribers remain healthy and out of hospitals. So, in a nutshell an *insurance company can stay afloat when it has large number of subscribers (which means lots of money coming in) and most of the subscribers remain healthy (which means lesser money going out).*

This means that as the insurance coverage increases, we as practicing doctors would be incentivized firstly to build and have our own Cohort or patient base and incentivized more to keep our cohort of patients healthy and out of hospitals. This is in total contrast to the prevailing conditions and business models that are geared up to push more people into hospitals. In the consumption versus connect spectrum, the healthcare industry will surely be forced to shift towards the connect side of the spectrum. (Please refer chapter 2).

Currently India is a young nation with an average age of around 29 years. Over 61 Crore Indians are below the age of 24 years of age and just about 9.5 crore Indians are above the age of 65 years of age [5]. Yet one and four Indians is at risk for non-communicable diseases and 60% of deaths are because of noncommunicable diseases. With passing time, the average age of population is going to increase. So, if the current trend continues the overall disease burden will be many times the current burden, and consequently, the expenditure on health care is bound to skyrocket. That is really bad. If you are an insurance company, your claims are going to go off the roof. To maintain the profit margins, you'll have to increase the premiums, which will definitely deter a large chunk of people from buying or renewing their health insurance and this will again stress out their profit margins setting in a vicious cycle of payor collapse.

Government of India and its think tanks are totally cognizant of these facts and are working relentlessly in this direction. The recent policy document by national health authority on value-based healthcare is a clear effort in this direction. Recent Government of India release in PIB (Press Information Bureau) mention the beginning of value-based healthcare in Ayushmann Bharat-PMJAY scheme. NHA is going to measure the value of healthcare services by measuring 5 broad parameters [6]. These parameters may not appear much but is certainly a very good start. Very soon we will certainly see many other finer and intricate parameters like clinical outcomes, mortality rates, morbidity rates, longitudinal health status etc coming in. This would require a robust technology infrastructure that can collect, analyze and improvise based on real-time data.

That brings us to the next big change factor which is flow of information. Ayushmann Bharat Digital Mission (ABDM) is one of the four pillars of Ayushmann Bharat Yojana. ABDM is aimed at creating a UHI (Universal Health Interface) which is supposed to replicate the thumping success of UPI (Unified Payment Interface). Essentially Government of India is trying to create a digital ecosystem where each Indian will have just one unique Health ID and with this ID she/he can find and access any health care professional or any health care facility without having to worry about carrying all their medical records every single time. It is aimed at creating a seamless experience for patients without any barrier. So why should we practicing doctors bother to know about these developments? Let's understand how UPI grew and revolutionized digital payments and that will help us predict what ABDM or UHI can do for us.

Digital payments in the form of mobile recharges and e-wallets have been around for almost 15 years now. Paytm started in the year 2010 and is one of the early birds. Back then paytm, freecharge and their likes operated in silos. That means if you wanted to transfer money to a shopkeeper, or your friend even they had to have the same app. If you used Paytm and your friend used freecharge, there was no way you could send them money. Each of these companies sweat it out to acquire users. They were largely seen as some hi-fi Tech Stuff that was used by mostly college going teenagers who were keen on cashbacks and discounts.

Then came demonetization in the year 2016, which practically forced the common man to adopt digital payments. Paytm use this opportunity to the hilt and made its presence felt with a huge user base. Government agencies had strategically launched UPI few months before demonetization. UPI provides a single interface through which you can send or receive money from anyone who also has a UPI ID, irrespective of which app both of you are using. You could be using Google Pay, the shopkeeper maybe using BharatPe and your friend maybe using PhonePe. Nevertheless, you can transfer and receive money from all of them without the hassle of downloading multiple apps.

As UPI started gaining traction with a boost from demonetization, e-wallets like Paytm appeared more cumbersome because you could send or receive money only from people who used Paytm. Paytm took a while to leverage UPI. However, new players like PhonePe, Bharathpe and Google pay cashed in on this big time and captured a large segment of users from Paytm which can be seen from the current market share of these companies in UPI transactions. PhonePe leads with 47% market share despite starting five years after Paytm started, Google pay has around 34% and Paytm around 15% of the total UPI transaction value [7].

How did this happen? It's simple, for someone who was using Paytm wallet, once they get a taste of convenience in UPI, it only takes two minutes to download google pay, PhonePe or any other app and start using it. To top it up, the new entrants gave out heavy cashbacks to acquire these customers. Common users like us would probably have downloaded two or more of these apps, depending on when and how much cash backs and discounts we got. This is known as the cashback war in the fin-tech lingo wherein these companies continue to bleed cash just to retain their customers. We learnt about this from a case study published by Think School in their youtube channel. (They are not specific to healthcare and cover general business case studies. These guys are amazing. You should check them out!).

Before UPI, the fin-tech companies had to just worry about acquiring customers and then making money by selling other products to this customer base. But after UPI, they have an additional challenge, they first need spend heavily to acquire customers and then work really hard to retain the same customers in order to make money by selling other products and services to the same customers. Since the walls are now broken, they're all finding innovative "retainer strategies" to safeguard their customer base.

Now let's compare this with ABDM/UHI. Once ABDM catches up, something very similar is going to happen in healthcare. Currently hospitals, nursing homes and clinics are operating in silos just like e-wallet used to operate before UPI. With UHI, these silos will break down. Just like user can switch to new UPI apps in barely couple of minutes, UHI will also enable the patients to find and switch to another app, hospital, nursing home or health care facility in a matter of minutes. This can be a potential challenge to the corporate hospital chains who are already struggling to retain their patient base. This could practically decimate the aggregators who are already burning cash to acquire customers and badly struggling to retain them.

Let's take for example I order online lab tests from say 1MG, I would prefer to go back to 1MG to repeat the test because my previous reports are in the same app. But with ABDM/UHI, I can switch to any other app say Netmeds, Lal Path, thyrocare or even my local neighborhood labs and get my blood tests done, without having to worry about losing my old test reports. Besides, we have already discussed the strong hyper-local nature of health care with the informal sector already dominating. ABDM/ UHI can create retention challenge for aggregators and corporate chains alike. They would need a very strong patient retainer strategy to sustain. The Human Nudge or HuDGE is practically their only solution.

Being aware of these revolutionary changes beforehand gives us an edge. We can gear up, utilize this opportunity and ride the wave. These upcoming changes are a huge blessing for practicing doctors like us, because whatever barriers were being created by certain market forces are going to be brought down. All we need to do is develop a strong HuDGE and my dear friends, rest of the healthcare industry will be at our doorsteps.

CHAPTER 12

Let's HuDGE

"An ounce of action is worth a ton of theory."

– Ralph Waldo Emerson

"Doctors with strong HuDGE will replace the Doctors without HuDGE"

It's time to

Break barriers

Build bridges

Bring benefits

Let's HuDGE!!!

Scan the QR Code or visit us at <u>www.navik.health</u>

References

Chapter 1:

1. "Health workforce in India: where to invest, how much and why?" Report by WHO and PFHI. Available at: https://www.who.int/publications/i/item/9789290209935

2. Karan A, Negandhi H, Hussain S, Zapata T, Mairembam D, De Graeve H, Buchan J, Zodpey S. Size, composition and distribution of health workforce in India: why, and where to invest?. Human resources for health. 2021 Dec;19(1):1-4.

3. https://scroll.in/article/1029766/how-true-is-the-health-ministers-claim-that-indias-doctor-population-ratio-exceeds-who-guidelines#:~:text=The%20latest%20National%20Sample%20Survey,approximately%204%25%20are%20unemployed%20and

4. PIB Release ID: 1796435 dated 8th February 2022, available at: https://pib.gov.in/PressReleaseIframePage.aspx?PRID=1796435

5. https://www.ibef.org/industry/healthcare-india

6. https://www.hdfcergo.com/blogs/health-insurance/medical-inflation-and-its-causes#:~:text=Current%20medical%20inflation%20rates%20in%20India&text=In%20FY%202022%2C%20while%20the,an%20overall%20growth%20of%2025%25.

Chapter 3:

1. https://www-ndtv-com.cdn.ampproject.org/c/s/www.ndtv.com/india-news/due-to-commercialisation-and-overburdened-healthcare-system-mistrust-and-suspicion-on-medical-services-becoming-narratives-chief-justice-of-india--dy-c-3816776/amp/1

Chapter 4:

1. Ramaswamy A, Gowda NR, Vikas H, Prabhu M, Sharma DK, Gowda PR, Mohan D, Kumar A. It's the data, stupid: Inflection point for Artificial Intelligence in Indian healthcare. Artificial Intelligence in Medicine. 2022 Jun 1;128:102300.

2. "Human Resources and Infrastructure for Health Sector in India": Report of Sub-Group-IV of Expert Committee on Enhancing Resource Investment in Health (ECERIH). Available on: https://nhsrcindia.org/sites/default/files/2021-06/20.Report%20of%20Sub%20Group%20IV%20of%20Expert%20Committee%20on%20enhancing%20resource%20investment%20in%20health.pdf

3. HDFC Securities Retail Research on Diagnostic Sector. Available on: https://www.hdfcsec.com/hsl.research.pdf/Diagnostics%20Sector%20-%20Initiating%20Coverage%20v2%20-%2030.03.2021.pdf

4. https://economictimes.indiatimes.com/prime/prime-vantage/as-pandemic-wave-recedes-heres-

what-is-holding-back-growth-of-diagnostic-companies/primearticleshow/96947360.cms

5. Sahu, Anupam, H. Vikas, and Nishant Sharma. "Life cycle costing of MRI machine at a tertiary care teaching hospital." *Indian Journal of Radiology and Imaging* 30.02 (2020): 190-194. Available on: https://www.ncbi.nlm.nih.gov/pmc/articles/PMC7546299/

6. Singh, Ankit, Priya Ravi, and Soniya Joseph. "A Comprehensive Break Even Analysis of MRI and CT Unit of a Tertiary Care Hospital in Sikkim." Indian Journal of Public Health Research & Development 11.3 (2020): 47-52.

7. https://www.medicalbuyer.co.in/government-the-savior-of-mri-market-2/

8. https://www.patientcentra.com/patient-recruitment-insights/clinical-trials-recruitment-social-media

9. https://vertassets.blob.core.windows.net/download/64c39d7e/64c39d7e-c643-457b-aec2-9ff7b65b3ad2/rdprecruitmentwhitepaper.pdf

10. https://www.ibef.org/industry/indian-pharmaceuticals-industry-analysis-presentation

11. https://www.nishithdesai.com/fileadmin/user_upload/pdfs/Research_Papers/Clinical-Trials-in-India.pdf

12. https://economictimes.indiatimes.com/industry/healthcare/biotech/pharmaceuticals/why-mnc-pharma-companies-are-realigning-their-india-operations/articleshow/89757660.cms?from=mdr

Chapter 5:

1.   https://stockanalysis.com/stocks/googl/statistics/

2.   https://www.statista.com/statistics/633651/alphabet-annual-global-revenue-by-segment/

3.   https://www.businessinsider.in/tech/news/googles-management-has-reportedly-issued-a-code-red-amid-the-rising-popularity-of-the-chatgpt-ai/articleshow/96407949.cms

4.   https://economictimes.indiatimes.com/tech/technology/google-bets-on-strong-ad-revenue-growth-in-india/articleshow/96434269.cms?from=mdr

5.   Press Information Bureau (PIB Release ID: 1884072) dated 16th December 2022. Available on: https://pib.gov.in/PressReleasePage.aspx?PRID=1884072

6.   OECD Going Digital Toolkit. Available on: https://goingdigital.oecd.org/dimension/use

7.   https://economictimes.indiatimes.com/tech/ites/dollar-fight-indian-youtubers-lag-in-global-earnings/articleshow/78307964.cms?from=mdr

8.   https://www.statista.com/statistics/237962/online-advertising-spending-in-india/

9.   Li X, Berger PD. MARKETING IN WESTERN VERSUS EASTERN CULTURE–COMPARING AND CONTRASTING BETWEEN THE US AND JAPAN. Journal of Research in Business, Economics and Management. 2018;11(3):2179-85.

10. https://www.livemint.com/news/india/as-downloads-surge-app-makers-in-india-struggle-to-retain-users-11613116393480.html

11. https://www.businessofapps.com/guide/mobile-app-retention/

12. https://www.statista.com/statistics/259329/ios-and-android-app-user-retention-rate/

13. https://www.shiprocket.in/blog/ten-amazon-statistics-in-2022/

14. https://www.businessofapps.com/marketplace/push-notifications/research/push-notifications-statistics/

Chapter 8:

1. https://www.ibef.org/blogs/india-emerging-as-a-medical-tourism-hub

2. "Human Resources and Infrastructure for Health Sector in India": Report of Sub-Group-IV of Expert Committee on Enhancing Resource Investment in Health (ECERIH). Available on: https://nhsrcindia.org/sites/default/files/2021-06/20.Report%20of%20Sub%20Group%20IV%20of%20Expert%20Committee%20on%20enhancing%20resource%20investment%20in%20health.pdf

3. Ramaswamy A, Gowda NR, Vikas H, Prabhu M, Sharma DK, Gowda PR, Mohan D, Kumar A. It's the data, stupid: Inflection point for Artificial Intelligence in Indian healthcare. Artificial Intelligence in Medicine. 2022 Jun 1;128:102300.

4. Anjali R, Gowda NR, Vikas H, Prabhu M, Sharma JB, Vakharia K, Kumar A, Akhila MV, Gatta S, Sareddy M, Sowmya KP. Out of Adversity Comes Opportunity: Smart-Colpo National Program for the Elimination of Carcinoma Cervix in a Post–COVID-19 World. Iproceedings. 2023 Mar 13;9(1):e41571.

Chapter 9:

1. https://www.ptinews.com/news/legal/delhi-hc-seeks-centres-stand-on-plea-for-action-against-health-service-aggregators/479846.html

2. https://www.shiprocket.in/blog/ten-amazon-statistics-in-2022/

3. https://www.investindia.gov.in/team-india-blogs/e-pharmacies-bridging-gap-indian-healthcare

Chapter 10:

1. https://www.youtube.com/watch?v=45PrXujlQCo

Chapter 11:

1. PIB Release ID: 1897272. Available on: https://www.pib.gov.in/PressReleasePage.aspx?PRID=1897272

2. https://www.youtube.com/watch?v=45PrXujlQCo

3. NITI Aayog report on "Health Insurance for India's Missing Middle". Available on: https://www.niti.gov.in/sites/default/files/2021-10/HealthInsurance-forIndiasMissingMiddle_28-10-2021.pdf

4. https://indianexpress.com/article/business/india-dependence-foreign-nations-health-care-narendra-modi-8481463/

5. https://ourworldindata.org/age-structure

6. PIB Release ID: 1889730 dated 9th January 2023. Available on: https://pib.gov.in/PressReleseDetailm.aspx?PRID=1889730

7. https://inc42.com/buzz/with-96-share-phonepe-google-pay-paytm-dominated-upi-transaction-count-in-december/#:~:text=%3D%223%22%5D-,With%2096%25%20Share%2C%20PhonePe%2C%2-0Google%20Pay%20%26%20Paytm%20Dominated,UPI%20Transaction%20Count%20In%20December&text=PhonePe%20and%20Google%20Pay%20continued,largest%20chunk%20of%20UPI%20transactions

Acknowledgement

The authors acknowledge the usefulness of generative AI tools like Bing, DALL-E and ideogram ai. They were used for creative illustrations in this book.